TOPICS IN AUTISM

Functional Behavior Assessment for People with Autism

MAKING SENSE OF SEEMINGLY SENSELESS BEHAVIOR

BETH A. GLASBERG, PH.D.

Sandra L. Harris, Ph.D., series editor

Woodbine House ◆ 2006

All rights reserved under International and Pan American copyright conventions.
Published in the United States of America by Woodbine House, Inc., 6510 Bells Mill
Road, Bethesda, MD 20817. 800-843-7323. www.woodbinehouse.com

Library of Congress Cataloging-in-Publication Data

Glasberg, Beth A.
  Functional behavior assessment for people with autism : making
sense of seemingly senseless behavior / by Beth A. Glasberg. -- 1st
ed.
     p. cm. -- (Topics in autism)
  Includes bibliographical references and index.
  ISBN-13: 978-1-890627-58-4
  ISBN-10: 1-890627-58-5
  1. Autism. 2. Autism in children. 3. Behavioral assessment.
4. Behavioral assessment of children. 5. Behavior disorders in
children.   I. Title. II. Series.
  RC553.A88G63 2005
  618.92'85882--dc22
                                                              2005019916

Manufactured in the United States of America

First edition

10 9 8 7 6 5 4 3

For Pete,

who somehow manages to tolerate

all of my seemingly senseless behaviors,

and for Spencer and Tessa,

who are so precious and make me so happy

that I never mind managing theirs.

Table of Contents

Acknowledgements

Just as it takes a village to raise a child, it takes a village to write a book as well. I'd like to acknowledge some of those villagers for their invaluable contributions.

First of all, I am indebted to Susan Stokes at Woodbine House for sharing her gift of practicality with this text. She transforms ideas into useful and readable writing. I am grateful for her support and consider it a privilege to be published by a company so committed to improving the lives of individuals with disabilities.

I have also been lucky to have had the opportunity to be mentored through my career by Sandra Harris. Her wisdom and grace provide a model to strive for, while her continual availability and support helps me along the road in pursuing my professional goals.

I'd also like to thank Lee Kern for introducing me to functional assessment. She helped create an opportunity for me to learn, and as a result changed the way that I think about behavior.

While much of the content of this book grows from what I've read in a book or journal, the majority of it grows out of experience. These experiences would not have been possible without the collaboration of the many families and educators who have shared their children and students with me. Many of you may recognize snippets of your own children in these pages. I thank you for your trust and partnership.

Also, I am eternally grateful to my own family. I literally could never have done this without Pete's support, help, love, laughter, and friendship. And a special thank you to Spencer and Tessa, who put a smile in my heart every day.

Last but not least, thanks to my Mom for being my test-reader and for calling periodically to get me on schedule, and to Mom and Nooch for doing my family's laundry once in a while so that I could get some work done! And, thanks to my Dad for temporarily suppressing his amazement that I could write a book without him.

Introduction

Is This Your Child?

Does your child engage in a behavior that just doesn't seem to make any sense? For example, does his behavior hurt or disturb others, or appear to go against what your child wants for himself? As a parent or teacher of someone displaying these seemingly senseless behaviors, you might find yourself feeling frustrated and confused. You are not alone. Unfortunately, these behaviors are fairly common among individuals with autism spectrum disorders. Take a look at the four stories below and see if any of them sound like your story.

Grace Carmichael

By October, Ms. Brandt was ready to quit her job. While she had thoroughly enjoyed teaching her second grade class for the last several years, this year was different. Little Grace Carmichael was ruining her life. Grace was an eight-year-old girl with a pervasive developmental disorder (PDD) who was included in Ms. Brandt's regular education classroom. Grace was very interested in other children and repeatedly told her mother how excited she was to be in her new classroom and to make friends. Grace might go days with no problems at all, and then suddenly, she might stand up, pick up her chair, and smash it on the foot of the child seated next to her. While doing a crafts activity, she might bite the arm of a student working with her. While standing in line, she might slap the child in front of her.

Grace's victims would yell at her or try to hit her back, but Grace persisted in her aggressive behavior. Grace had been sent to the principal's office, lost her dessert at lunchtime, and had her mother called to come and pick her up—all to no avail; the behaviors persisted. Ms. Brandt wanted to help Grace, but she had virtually no experience with special education or behavior problems. The consulting special education teacher had never worked with behavior problems this inconsistent or severe. Although Grace was making progress in her academics, socially her classroom placement was a failure. The other children had become afraid of her. Ms. Brandt felt bad about asking to place Grace in a more restrictive setting because she felt that Grace had the potential to benefit from the inclusive setting, but she believed that these dangerous and disruptive behaviors were leaving her no choice.

Jamaal Brown's Story

Four-year-old Jamaal Brown had been doing so well in his home-based discrete trial instruction program that his parents and teachers were starting to eye the mainstream kindergarten classroom as a possible placement for the upcoming school year. Not only was he flying through his academic, self-help, and motor programs, but his social skills programming was also going swimmingly. He could have entire conversations about various topics while using appropriate body language and intonation. His parents and teachers were sure he was ready for typically developing peers, and enrolled Jamaal in a children's gymnastics class to see how he would do. Much to their surprise, Jamaal did not interact well with the other children. Although he watched them closely and seemed interested in their activities, he did not approach them. When peers approached him, Jamaal would look right at them while making a strange face and adopting a crooked posture with his body. Sadly, the other children quickly stopped trying to play with Jamaal.

Darra Littman

If Darra Littman's mother had told her once, she had told her a thousand times: no more discussion of pop singer Clay Aiken. Darra had seen Clay on the American Idol television show and hadn't stopped talking about him since. At first, Darra's parents were excited—finally, their daughter with Asperger's disorder was interested in an age-appropriate icon. The embarrassment of having a preteen who adored Sesame Street characters was at last at an end. And her peers noticed! They were very impressed with Darra's knowledge of all things "Clay."

Unfortunately, Darra's interest in Clay continued to mushroom. She began to turn almost any conversation his direction, no matter how unrelated. These odd changes of topic made her peers uncomfortable and eventually resulted in them avoiding her. Nevertheless, Darra's focus on Clay intensified. She could discuss nothing else. At this point, her mother decided to end the obsessive talk. She forbade any discussion of Clay. Furthermore, she made a rule that any mention of his name would cost Darra ten minutes of evening television time, which Darra treasured. Nevertheless, the "Clay" talk persisted. Last night, Darra lost all two hours of her allotted television time in the evening. The strange part was, this had no discernable impact on the "Clay" talk. Mrs. Littman could not understand why this behavior was so out of control.

Anthony Cappozolli

Mr. Cappozolli heard that familiar, unwelcome sound in the living room and went running. Just as he'd expected, he found Anthony, his nonverbal, fifteen-year-old son with autism, banging his head against the windowpane. "Anthony!" he yelled, pulling him away. He sternly reminded him that head banging is dangerous and not allowed. Mr. Cappozolli then led Anthony over to a box of beads, off limits at other times, that the family used to distract him from continuing this perilous behavior.

Today, the Cappozollis were lucky—Anthony hadn't broken the glass. Other times, they had not been so lucky. This behavior had cost them numerous trips to the emergency room and numerous window-

panes. More importantly, it had cost Anthony's parents an untold amount of worry and grief, and had given them a sickening sense that they were helpless to protect their own son from himself. While grateful that he and his wife had the beads to interrupt the head banging, Mr. Cappozolli wished that he could understand where the head banging came from, and ultimately prevent it altogether.

The four children described above illustrate just a few of the behavior problems that children with an autism spectrum disorder may display. Your child may be challenging you with noncompliance, inattention, repetitive behaviors, or other problems. Some behaviors may be life-threatening, while others are just plain irritating. Some behaviors may lead to the destruction of property, while others may lead to the destruction of relationships with family or friends. For some parents, these behaviors are a constant, painful reminder of their child's disability. For others, they may be a constant barrier to getting their child into the community and participating in the world.

While each type of behavior appears very different from the others, they do share a common thread. Each of the above behaviors does not seem to make any sense. The children engaging in these behaviors are losing things they value, ranging from television time to positive interactions with peers, but they are engaging in the behaviors anyway. Some behaviors, such as Anthony's head banging, appear to be enormously painful, yet the behaviors persist. For those who care about these children and desperately want them to be safe, happy individuals with a rich circle of friends and loved ones, these behaviors are enormously frustrating and are often the barriers between where these children are and where we want them to be. The purpose of this book is to help tear down these barriers. This book will help readers to identify how and why these troubling behaviors arise as well as to learn the basics of a strategy to eliminate them. Additionally, while this book cannot help with certain behaviors that require medication (such as tics), it can help you learn to distinguish behaviors that are part of underlying medical issues from those that will respond to behavioral intervention.

Over the years, research and experience have taught professionals who study behavior that making sense of a seemingly senseless behavior is an essential step to controlling it. This means that we must accept that these behaviors make perfect sense to the individuals engaging in them and then identify why. We must ask ourselves, "What purpose is this behavior serving?" and "How is this behavior benefiting my child?"

Well-established procedures have been developed to systematically identify the factors contributing to the occurrence of behavior problems in people with disabilities. Collectively, these procedures are referred to as "functional behavior assessment." Results of functional behavior assessments are then ideally used to develop effective behavior intervention plans.

Study after study shows that relying on a thorough functional behavior assessment is the most likely way to succeed in addressing an unwanted behavior (e.g., Repp, Felce, & Barton, 1988). Behavior intervention plans based on functional behavior assessments work for individuals of all ages and all functioning levels (e.g., Austin, Weatherly, & Gravina, 2005; Ervin, DuPaul, Kern, & Friman, 1998; Hanley, Piazza, Fisher, & Maglieri, 2005). This approach is relevant for the most severely impaired individuals with a dual diagnosis of autism and mental retardation as well as for typically developing children and adults with no diagnosis at all. The research behind functional behavior assessment is so compelling that legally, public schools in the United States *must* consider completing this type of assessment when addressing challenging behaviors (Individuals with Disabilities Education Act, 2004).

You do not have to be an expert in behavior analysis to understand and implement a functional behavior assessment. This book will teach readers how to complete comprehensive functional behavior assessments independently. It is written to help parents, grandparents, group home staff, and other caregivers, as well as teachers, school psychologists, and other professionals who may not have had access to specific training in this area. The methods described in this book can be used with toddlers, preschoolers, school-aged children, adolescents, and adults with any type of autism spectrum disorder, as well as other individuals with problem behaviors.

A general introduction to the principles of behavior will be provided in Chapters 1 and 2, including a discussion of how challenging behaviors arise and why individuals with autism spectrum disorders are more susceptible to developing them. Other foundation topics covered in these chapters will include an introduction to the principles of learning, a discussion of factors determining which behaviors will be performed in a given situation, and an overview of the types of consequences that may strengthen behaviors. Furthermore, Chapter 1 includes an overview of functional behavior assessment and a discussion of how functional behavior assessment helps make sense of otherwise perplexing behaviors. This background will equip readers for Chapters 3 through 8, which together present a practical, step-by-step guide to completing a functional assessment, including "Keep it Simple Tips" to make the process more manageable, and handy tools to use when completing an assessment. This guide will help readers learn how to interpret assessment results, which are ultimately needed to develop an effective intervention. Finally, Chapter 9 will cover special topics such as adult issues, very infrequent but severe behaviors, and troubleshooting.

Armed with this combination of knowledge and skills, the reader will then be ready to make sense of those seemingly senseless behaviors and help their child or student tear down barriers to leading fuller and happier lives. If someone you care about is being held back by interfering behaviors, you can gain the skills to make a difference in their lives. To begin empowering yourself to help, read on.

1 | Why Problem Behaviors Occur

Most problem behaviors are puzzling. Think about the examples described in the Introduction. Why would Anthony inflict so much pain on himself? Why would Grace destroy her chances of friendship with such violent behaviors? The answers to these questions are just not obvious. Professionals have struggled to understand behavior problems for a very long time. This chapter will give you a quick overview of how our thinking about the causes of, and interventions for, behavior problems has changed over time, and then tie that into the current thinking about why problem behaviors occur so often in individuals with autism spectrum disorders (ASDs).

How Do We Think about Behavior Problems? A Quick History

Historically, behavior interventions did not take into account the possible causes for a behavior. Instead, they focused on the question, "What is she doing?" Based on what a behavior looked like and what body parts were involved, a punishment was chosen. For example, if a boy swore, his mother might wash his mouth out with soap. If a girl with autism hit someone, her teacher might hold her arms down at her side for thirty seconds. Through a trial and error process using this strategy, caregivers looked for an effective punishment. In fact, a punishment-based approach, such as this one, is often the first intervention strategy that many nonprofessionals try even today.

There are numerous problems with this approach. First of all, when we use this type of punishment, we never find out what the individual has been gaining from performing the problem behavior. The fact that she did it at all tells us that she was getting something out of it. Therefore, even if our punishment works, meaning that it gets rid of the behavior, the individual still has no appropriate way to get what she wants. This makes it likely that she will find a new way to meet her need—and we may not like it any better than the old way. For example, if a boy is punished for hitting his teacher whenever he is asked to do his schoolwork, he may indeed stop hitting her, but start swiping work materials off of his desk instead. Either behavior will have the equivalent effect of postponing his schoolwork.

Secondly, if we take action without knowing what the child has been getting out of a behavior, we may inadvertently reward it. Let's revisit the boy who was hitting his teacher. For this example, let's imagine that this behavior persisted because it helped him avoid his work. If we punish him by sending him to the principal's office (away from his work), we are inadvertently rewarding his behavior and increasing the chances that he will hit again.

A final problem with this type of punishment is that an individual may "habituate," or get used to, a certain level of punishment over time (e.g., Ratner, 1970). This requires the person doing the intervention to gradually increase the intensity of the punishment in order to maintain its effectiveness. For example, the first time that you want your son to stop poking his sister, you may be able to deter him with a stern voice. Over time, you may need to raise your voice a bit. Soon, you may find yourself actually yelling, and so on. Eventually, you may arrive at some level of punishment that you are not comfortable with. When you consider escalation of other forms of punishment, from putting something that tastes bad into a child's mouth up through spanking, you can see how the need for increased intensity becomes more and more problematic.

A second intervention for difficult behaviors that has historically been very popular and remains very popular is "time-out" (Ferster, 1958). There are various permutations of time-out procedures, but the most basic element of this intervention is the removal of an individual from the setting where the behavior problem occurred. For example, a student who hits in class may be removed from the classroom for a given period of time. Time-out offers an alternative to more traditional, physical forms of punishment-based discipline, such as spanking, and is firmly entrenched in current parenting culture. Stop any parent at your local playground and ask how long a time-out for a five-year-old should be. They will likely inform you, without a moment's hesitation, to use one minute for every year of the child's age. Parents and teachers everywhere have become time-out experts.

Despite its celebrity, there are problems with relying on time-out as the solution to every behavior problem. In fact, at times, using time-out actually might encourage a child to engage in a behavior more often. For example, in 1994, Brian Iwata and his colleagues summarized their work with over 150 people with developmental disabilities who were hurting themselves, a classic example of a seemingly senseless behavior. The research revealed that almost 40 percent of the time, self-injury was occurring as a way of getting out of or away from something. As with our example above of the boy who hit to escape work, these individuals were hurting themselves in an effort to leave a situation. As you might imagine, if a child who engaged in self-injury was sent to time-out, then we would see a cycle in which the child is motivated to escape a situation, hurts herself, and escapes the situation. This would lead to more, rather than less, self-injury in the future.

Another challenge associated with time-out is that many children require a great deal of intervention to get them to their time-out location. This intervention may take the form of repeated instructions to go to time-out, hand holding while walking to the time-out area, or more involved physical guidance. Each of these strategies is associated with a high level of attention. If a child is engaging in a problem behavior in order to get attention, time-out may actually lead to rewarding the inappropriate behavior.

Current Thinking about the Purpose of Challenging Behavior

In the 1980s, there was a shift in the field of behavioral psychology toward viewing problematic behaviors as a form of communication. To change behaviors, we now focus on the question, "What message is that behavior communicating?" rather than on what the behavior looks like. We now know that even the most seemingly senseless behaviors make sense for the person performing the behavior.

Problematic behaviors are learned in the same manner as other forms of communication: an individual who has some need identifies a behavior to get his need met. The example above illustrates this: The boy who learned that hitting his instructor resulted in the removal of his work communicated, "Take away my work, please" by hitting. Other consequences, such as getting his hands held down by his sides or getting a talking-to from the principal, do not prevent him from learning this communication. What matters for him at that moment is that he is motivated to escape his work, and, as a result of hitting or swiping materials off of the table, he does.

Research done by Ted Carr and Mark Durand (1985) was instrumental in developing this clearer understanding of behavior problems. They documented predictable relationships between problem behaviors and the individual's environment. For example, certain people would display their problem behaviors only when they were receiving very little attention. Others might display their problem behaviors whenever they were given a very difficult task to do. Different individuals displayed their problem behaviors under different conditions. The same behavior in two different individuals might be elicited by two very different sets of conditions. By demonstrating these relationships, Carr and Durand helped to teach us that what a behavior looks like tells us very little about its origin or how to treat it.

A real-life illustration of Carr and Durand's work is provided by the behaviors of two teenage boys, Andrew and Robert. Consultation was requested for each of the boys for the same reason, aggression. Andrew blocked the door whenever a one-to-one pull-out teaching session, such as speech or counseling, was ending. He then poked his teacher if she tried to leave the room. If the staff member persisted in attempting to leave, Andrew upped the ante by threatening to hit her with scissors or to hit her with a telephone. Further assessment of this behavior revealed that Andrew behaved this way in order to maintain the rich, one-to-one attention that he had access to during these supportive therapies.

Like Andrew, Robert also poked people. Whenever his siblings sat near him or walked close enough, a swat or a poke was guaranteed. However, a closer look at Robert's behavior revealed a story very different from Andrew's. Robert poked people in order to make them go away. The longer they stayed, the more forceful the poking and swatting became. As you might imagine, Robert's siblings learned very quickly to stay away from him. A particularly exciting result of this study was that Carr and Durand were also able to show that teaching and reinforcing an appropriate request for whatever was desired weakened the problem behaviors. The success of this approach, referred to as "functional communication training," clearly demonstrates that the difficult behaviors so often displayed by individuals with autism spectrum disorders are not an automatic byproduct of the disorder, but rather are learned behaviors, open to treatment using all of the principles of learning.

Other researchers have experimented not only with conditions that might set the stage for a problem behavior, but also with conditions that they suspected might follow a problem behavior (Iwata, Dorsey, Slifer, Bauman, & Richman, 1982). This research helped demonstrate that what happens before a behavior can create a motivation for something and that engaging in a problem behavior can result in obtaining what is wanted. To illustrate, consider the boy in our example above: the teacher approaching his desk with work materials created a motivation for him to be someplace else. Hitting his teacher resulted in him being sent to the principal's office, thereby avoiding his work. The consequences of the behavior were critical to the development of the behavior problem.

Brian Iwata and his colleagues (1982) demonstrated this idea empirically. They placed people in scenarios that mimicked these supposedly naturally occurring conditions and measured the effect on their behavior. For example, they might withhold attention from a study participant while she played with toys, but then provide attention when she performed the problem behavior (self-injury). Upon the occurrence of self-injury, the experimenter would immediately return his attention to the girl in the form of social disapproval (e.g., "Don't do that; you'll hurt yourself!"). When the consequences for the behavior were presented consistently in this way, the researchers were able to reliably produce stable patterns of the problem behavior. Using this counterintuitive approach, the researchers replicated what they believed was taking place in the real world and leading to learning. Their results showed that their hypothesis was correct: the study participants were learning these problem behaviors based on their consequences.

Iwata and his colleagues also identified a special kind of behavior that is learned through internal cues and consequences. These behaviors occur because they feel good or are inherently enjoyable for the person performing them. The conditions that trigger these behaviors and the consequences that maintain them occur inside of the individual, and thus are more complex to assess or control. Everyday examples of this type of behavior might include scratching an itch or taking a pain reliever. An observer cannot see the itch or the headache, nor can she document the consequences of removal of the itch or the headache. However, these behaviors are learned based upon the same principles as externally controlled behaviors and numerous strategies exist to help address them.

By examining patterns of what happens before and after problem behaviors, Iwata and his colleagues were able to identify a number of communicative messages that challenging behaviors might convey. In other words, they identified the purposes that these behaviors were serving for the individuals performing them. These different purposes that behaviors serve are called "functions" of behavior and are described in Chapter 2. A quest to identify the functions of different problem behaviors was born, leading to the emergence of the field we know as "functional behavior assessment."

Why Are Problematic Behaviors So Common among Individuals with Autism Spectrum Disorders?

While all people, children and adults, typically developing or disabled, may have behavior problems, they are more common among individuals with autism spectrum disorders. When you think about the specific areas of disability associated with this group of disorders, the reasons for this relationship become clear.

Difficulties with Communication Skills

First of all, individuals with autism spectrum disorders often show impairments in communication. Consider Anthony, described in the Introduction. Recall that Anthony was nonverbal. Also recall that his family distracted him from head banging with a special box of beads. In order to keep the beads exciting for Anthony, his family had made the beads off-limits for him at other times. Therefore, Anthony was repeatedly exposed to the following sequence:

1. I have no beads.
2. I bang my head.
3. I get beads.

Anthony's head banging brings beads into his environment. Since Anthony lacks the communication skills to ask for the beads, he may have learned that banging his head is the best way for him to communicate a request for them. Even if he could request them some other way, they are off limits to him unless he is banging his head.

In a similar scenario, a colleague worked with one nonverbal student who engaged in aggressive behaviors so severe that numerous staff who worked with him had required medical attention for problems as serious as a broken nose. For safety reasons, each time he engaged in an aggressive behavior, he was restrained in a cushiony restraint on a soft mat. A functional behavior assessment revealed that his aggressions were actually his way of requesting access to this restraint. To reduce his aggression, he was given a picture card that he could use to request the restraint. Once he mastered this communication, his aggressive behaviors virtually disappeared.

This is not to say that individuals with ASDs who can speak or sign are immune from exhibiting problem behaviors. Some people can communicate but the skill is challenging enough for them that a problem behavior is simpler. For example, a child with communicative challenges who would like a break from her classwork faces two options:

1. Identify a cue from the teacher that it is okay to raise your hand, raise your hand, wait to be called on, formulate a sentence requesting a break, and wait to see whether the teacher says yes or no; or
2. Bang the materials on your desk loudly and get sent immediately to time-out. The latter behavior seems much more efficient for the child.

Difficulties with Social Skills

Individuals with autism spectrum disorders also have social skills deficits. This means they do not engage in social interaction as easily as other people. Similarly, they may not be as skilled at interpreting social responses from others. Therefore, any social reaction they elicit may be rewarding for them. Consider Grace, our second grader who was assaulting her peers. Lacking the skills to have more meaningful social interactions, Grace may settle for the yelling and hitting that her peers are doing in response to her aggression if she cannot elicit friendly responses.

I was called in to consult with teachers about a preschooler with autism who was exhibiting a similar behavior pattern. This child was a bit larger than the other students in his segregated preschool classroom and was also more interested in socializing than his classmates were. He would often try to approach them appropriately, but would get no response. He then moved on to "belly-bopping" them, bumping them roughly with his belly. Unfortunately, this inappropriate behavior was sure to get his classmates' attention. Although the attention was often in the form of crying or yelling, for the student exhibiting the behavior, this was preferable to no response at all. Despite his behavior problem, this child was transferred to an integrated preschool classroom where the other children were more socially aware. In this setting, where the other children responded to his more appropriate initiations, his "belly-bopping" disappeared without any other specific intervention.

Challenging behaviors can also stem from a desire to avoid or escape social contact. Think back to Jamaal, who made odd faces or adopted strange postures whenever his peers approached him. Jamaal's behavior quickly taught the other children to leave him alone and may have been Jamaal's way of asking them to go away. Although Jamaal's educational programming likely focused upon approaching other children and extending interactions, failing to teach children how to end or avoid social interactions is a common teaching oversight. Similarly, Robert, the teenager described above who swatted and poked his siblings to get them to keep their distance, could probably benefit from instruction in social skills for appropriately escaping interactions.

Restricted Interests

Finally, a restricted behavioral repertoire is associated with autism spectrum disorders. This means that children with ASDs have fewer areas of interest and may focus on parts of an object or activity, rather than the whole thing. This phenomenon has been described as viewing the world with a laser beam rather than a flashlight. Darra's interest in Clay Aiken, described in the Introduction, provides a good example of this keen focus. While other preteens may have a number of pop icons who consume their interest, Darra has only Clay. Additionally, other preteens may have topics other than pop icons that attract them, such as sports, dance, puzzles, books, etc. Darra's range of interests is not as broad.

This narrow range of interests is bound to lead to a variety of problems stemming from repetition. Rather than engaging in a variety of behaviors, the individual is doing the same thing over and over again. As for Darra, this hyper-focus may lead to social problems. She is like a record where the needle is stuck in a groove and keeps playing the same section of music. In other individuals, this constricted focus may play out as repetitive actions, such as hand flapping or rocking, which may be stigmatizing or even dangerous. The individual, stuck in a groove, is repeating the same behavior over and over.

Finally, some individuals may pursue their interests so single-mindedly that it leads to risky behaviors or an infringement on the rights of others. Darius McCollum, who has been diagnosed with Asperger's disorder, provides a famous example of this possibility. Darius grew up in New York City and always loved trains. He focused so intently on subways and commuter trains that he became knowledgeable enough to "steal" trains and subway cars by posing as the driver and making all of the correct stops. In fact, he has spent more than fifteen of his thirty-nine years in jail for these thefts. Furthermore, he reports that he has committed his crime far more often than he has been caught. Even being imprisoned has not been a deterrent for him. Sadly, only days before this writing, Darius pled guilty to another "train robbery" with a maximum three-year sentence for a crime he committed just months after his last prison release.

2 | How Are Behaviors Learned?

In the Introduction, we met four children: Jamaal, Darra, Grace, and Anthony, who each exhibited very different behavior problems. The commonality among their stories is that their behaviors don't seem to make any sense. If you are reading this book, you have probably also come across a perplexing behavior or two yourself.

The only way to develop an understanding of how these challenging behaviors were learned and actually do make sense is to develop an understanding of how behaviors are learned more generally. The following section will provide a tutorial of the most important aspects of learning theory to enable you to rely on this foundation when completing a functional behavior assessment. Because functional behavior assessment grows out of learning theory, this background is essential.

Beware—this will be by far the most technical section of the book. Don't let that scare you. Once you get the gist of the concepts described below, you will have a far clearer sense of behavior, which will make the rest of your days as a behavior interventionist significantly easier.

Overview of Learning Theory

Learning implies that a behavior is added to an individual's repertoire in a relatively permanent way (Catania, 1998). One can learn skills, such as addition and subtraction, or behaviors, such as brushing teeth or washing hands. One might also learn problem behaviors, such as head banging or endlessly discussing Clay Aiken. If learning were a mathematical equation it would look like this:

Motivation + Antecedent + Behavior + Consequence = Learning

In other words, learning is the sum of four variables. We will explore each of the four variables below. Although a consequence comes chronologically at the *end* of a learning sequence, the terms and concepts relevant to consequences are important to an understanding of the first three learning variables. Therefore, consequences will be discussed first.

1) Consequences

A consequence is what occurs as the result of a behavior. In general, a consequence can be …
1. reinforcement, or
2. punishment.

Reinforcement

Reinforcement involves consequences that strengthen behavior. To "strengthen a behavior" means to increase the likelihood that it will occur in the future, or to increase its intensity or duration in the future. Examples of reinforcement include a woman being told that a dress looks good on her, resulting in her wearing that dress very often; a child being given a quarter for cleaning his room, resulting in him cleaning it every day; or an infant discovering that his mobile will shake around if he kicks, resulting in him kicking his legs repeatedly. In these examples, specific behaviors are strengthened by their consequences.

There are two types of reinforcement procedures: positive reinforcement and negative reinforcement.

Positive Reinforcement. When "positive reinforcement" is at work, the consequence that strengthens behavior involves adding something to the individual's environment. For example, beads were added to Anthony's environment as a consequence for head banging. His parents had unintentionally delivered positive reinforcement for head banging. Positive reinforcement can involve receiving access to anything that the individual is motivated to obtain, including attention, a certain sensation, a particular activity, food, money, tokens, etc.

Some things that act as positive reinforcers don't look appealing to an outsider at all. For example, the "belly-bopper" described in Chapter 1 was getting tears and yells from peers and this consequence was strengthening his behavior of belly-bopping. Tears and yells were acting as positive reinforcers for belly bopping. The other student described in Chapter 1 was physically restrained when he was aggressive, and this consequence was strengthening his behavior of aggression. A physical restraint was acting as positive reinforcement for aggression.

The only way to determine whether a given consequence is a reinforcer is to measure its effect on behavior. If it increases a behavior, it's a reinforcer. Remember, reinforcers don't have to look good; they just have to strengthen behavior.

Here's a quick quiz:

1. If I give my son a Skittle every time he goes pee-pee in the potty, but he is doing it less and less, have I reinforced the behavior? No, because the consequence is decreasing the behavior.

2. If I yell every time my son goes in the potty and complain loudly that now I have to clean it out, and he goes more and more in the potty, have I reinforced the behavior? Yes, because this consequence is increasing the probability of pee-pee in the potty.

3. If I give my son a star on a chart every time he goes in the potty, have I reinforced the behavior? We don't know. It's a trick question. You can't tell because I haven't told you the effect on his behavior.

Negative Reinforcement. The second type of reinforcement procedure that is important to understand when addressing challenging behavior is "negative reinforcement." There are a lot of misconceptions surrounding this term. Many people think that negative reinforcement is equivalent to punishment. Others believe that negative reinforcement involves "negative attention" like scolding a child for misbehavior. In fact, the term "negative" does not imply an unpleasant consequence. Instead, it simply means that behavior is strengthened by *removing* something from someone's environment.

Everyday examples of behaviors strengthened by negative reinforcement include: hitting the snooze button on your alarm clock (removing the aversive sound of the alarm from your environment), putting sunglasses on (removing the aversive glare from your environment), or taking off shoes that are too tight (removing the painful sensation from your internal environment). The student described on page 2 who has learned to hit his teacher to escape his work illustrates a negative reinforcement procedure. When he hits his teacher, work gets removed from his environment, and he becomes more likely to hit again under similar circumstances in the future.

Let's try another quick quiz:

1. If I cross one homework assignment off a student's list for each minute that he participates in a group project, and he gradually participates in group for longer and longer periods of time, what type of procedure was this? Negative reinforcement (consequence = homework removed from the environment).

2. If peers laugh each time that Johnny makes a wisecrack at the teacher, and he makes more and more wisecracks, what type of procedure was this? Positive reinforcement (consequence = peer attention added to Johnny's environment).

3. If Johnny loses five minutes of recess each time he makes a wisecrack at the teacher, and he makes more and more wisecracks, what type of procedure was this? Negative reinforcement (consequence = recess—which to Johnny might mean difficult social demands and unstructured time—removed from his environment).

4. If Teresa earns a quarter toward the price of a movie ticket each time she washes the dishes at her group home and she volunteers for dish-washing duty more and more often, what type of procedure is this? Positive reinforcement (consequence = quarters added to Teresa's environment).

5. If I move farther away from a student who is uncomfortable with proximity each time that he screams, what type of procedure was this? This is another trick question; the effect on behavior wasn't mentioned.

Punishment

A second type of consequence that might follow a behavior is punishment. The specific consequence is technically referred to as a "punisher." A punisher is any consequence that decreases the strength (future probability, intensity, or duration) of a behavior. An example of a punisher is your spouse telling you, in a lukewarm tone, that you look "fine" in your carefully selected outfit. The future probability of your wearing that outfit will surely decrease. A school-based example of a punisher might involve assigning extra homework to a student as a consequence for disruptive behavior during the school day. If it decreases the future probability of the disruptive behavior, then this consequence is acting as a punisher.

Just as with reinforcement, there are positive and negative punishment procedures. In a positive punishment procedure, something is added to the environment (e.g., a lukewarm "fine" or extra homework) that weakens a behavior. The particular thing that is added to the environment leading to the decrease in behavior is sometimes referred to as an "aversive." In contrast, with a negative punishment procedure, something is removed from the environment, leading to a decrease in a behavior. For example, you might take car privileges away from your teenaged daughter for a specified period of time if she gets home past her curfew. In this case, the hope is that losing this valued privilege for a while will decrease the probability of her coming home late once her privileges are returned. Similarly, a child might lose ten minutes of television time for each disrespectful comment made to a teacher at school. The goal of this would be to decrease the future probability of disrespectful comments made to teachers. Generally speaking, items that might be effective as positive reinforcers are candidates to be removed as part of a negative punishment procedure (e.g., tokens toward a reward, privileges, etc.), as their loss will likely lead to a behavior change.

Like reinforcement, the term "punishment" is defined by its impact on behavior. Therefore, giving a student M&M's can actually be a punisher if it decreases a behavior, and yelling at him can actually be a reinforcer if it increases his behavior. It is only the effect on behavior that determines which procedure has taken place.

Keep It Simple Summary

1. A reinforcer strengthens (increases) behavior.
2. A punisher weakens (decreases) behavior.
3. The term "positive" means that something is added to the environment.
4. The term "negative" means that something is removed from the environment.

Consequence-Based Procedures

	Reinforcer	Punisher
Positive	Adding something strengthens behavior	Adding something weakens behavior
Negative	Taking away something strengthens behavior	Taking away something weakens behavior

2) *Motivation*

Motivation, in everyday language, refers to what a person wants or desires, as well as how hard he is willing to work to get it. For example, someone might be motivated to get out of work early for a long weekend or motivated to attain good grades in school.

In the study of behavior, the meaning of motivation is very close to this but with one major difference. In behavior analysis, we think of motivation in terms of external, measurable factors. When we think of motivation as something internal, as in the colloquial use of the word, that doesn't leave us any way to observe or control it. For example, if we say someone wants to get out of work early for a long weekend, we cannot measure how much he wants this. If we say that someone is motivated to attain good grades in school, we cannot directly increase or decrease this desire. Because motivation drives behavior, if we cannot measure or control it, we cannot change behavior. In the section below, we will describe a strategy developed by behavior analysts to quantify and alter motives.

Establishing Operations (EO's)

Led by the work of Jack Michael (1982), behavior analysts have developed a more quantifiable way to think about motivation referred to as "establishing operations" or EO's. You can think of these as "operations" on someone's environment that "establish" a motivation for certain items or events. To work with EO's, you observe or manipulate what an individual has had access to and draw conclusions about what might be motivating to him at any given moment. For example, while we can't watch a person and learn how hungry he is, we can observe the number of hours since he has last eaten and draw conclusions about how motivated he may be to get some food. Similarly, we cannot measure how much a person wants to get out of work early to start his vacation, but we can measure the number of hours since his last vacation.

Thinking about EO's also highlights the ever-changing nature of motivators. Consider this scenario: For a teen who hasn't eaten all day, pizza will certainly be an effective positive reinforcer for completing chores. In everyday language, we can say that the teen is motivated to eat. As behavior analysts, we can say that an EO for food is in effect. However, with every bite of pizza, the teen becomes less food-deprived, and therefore less motivated to eat more. Let's say our teen has now polished off a whole pizza. Offering pizza as a consequence for completing chores now will be unlikely to strengthen the behavior, and may even act as a punisher for completing chores. EO's help us understand the frustrating reality that the strongest motivator for your child one day will not necessarily be effective at all the next day.

Some readers may have seen this effect in their own experience. For example, a commonly used intervention for children with autism who have a behavior problem is a technique referred to as a DRO (differential reinforcement of other behavior). This technique involves offering the person a reward for every interval of time that passes when a specified problem behavior has not occurred. Sometimes an interval as brief as one minute may be used. Often, parents or teachers use the child's favorite treat for this procedure.

Not infrequently, a DRO may be wildly effective at first and then stop working. This often baffles the parents or teachers running the intervention. When we consider the impact of the EO on this situation, the reason becomes clear. Let's say someone who bites his own hand is on a one-minute DRO schedule earning M&M's. That means that every minute that passes without hand biting, he is given one M&M. After one hour, he has eaten 60 M&M's. After two hours, he has eaten 120 M&M's. After four hours, he has eaten 240 M&M's. As much as anyone enjoys M&M's, how many minutes will pass before he or she throws the bag of M&M's on the floor? Like the pizza, the M&M's that were initially reinforcing can also become a punisher.

The strength of an EO for any particular thing will be in constant flux. You can think of EO's as being on a continuum (see next page) from deprivation (too little) to satiation (too much). As time passes without access to something, the EO moves left on the continuum toward deprivation. As the individual enjoys more and more of something, the EO moves right on the continuum. EO's apply to everything in the environment, from basic needs such as food, drink, or temperature, to objects and activities such as a favorite toy or game. Different types of stimulation, such as music or touch, as well as social interaction of different types, such as speaking softly, intense reactions, or physical contact, are all subject to EO's.

Similarly, EO's apply to aversive stimuli, which may include loud noises, pain, noxious tastes or odors, etc. In this case, the individual will be motivated to move towards deprivation.

EO CONTINUUM

Deprivation ← → Satiation

EO's have two effects on behavior. The first is giving certain consequences the power to strengthen behavior. In other words, EO's establish reinforcers. For example, when Anthony's parents deprive him of access to his favorite beads, the beads become a potent reinforcer for any behavior that leads to playing with them (such as hitting his head against the window). The second effect of an EO is that it will often elicit behaviors that have led to reinforcement in the past. So, being deprived of his favorite beads for a certain period of time will often trigger head banging against the window for Anthony.

Remember, an EO is not always something tangible. For example, being deprived of music or social praise makes those consequences more reinforcing as well (Vollmer & Iwata, 1991). Sometimes we notice that children are more likely to engage in a problem behavior because they are "bored." A technical way to think of being bored might be deprivation of stimulation or preferred activities.

The amount of deprivation that will elicit a given behavior varies from person to person. You can think of this as a given individual's threshold. Whenever that threshold is reached, the target behavior will result. This threshold is ever-changing and is affected by remote events such as not getting enough sleep, fighting with your spouse in the morning, or feeling a little under the weather. For example, I may not typically be motivated to respond to someone cutting me off on the highway by yelling expletives to myself in the car (automatic reinforcement), but if I wake up late in the morning, rush to get ready only to be held up by the babysitter arriving late, stop for coffee anyway and discover the line is too long, and then get cut off on the highway, my threshold for motivation to perform that behavior is lower and it will take less external input before I start swearing.

For more information on EO's and people with autism, see *Incentives for Change: Motivating People with Autism Spectrum Disorders to Learn and Gain Independence* (Delmolino and Harris, 2004).

Keep It Simple Summary

EO's are a way to think about motivation. The more you are deprived of something desired—the more you will want it. You will try behaviors that have worked in the past to get it, and getting what you want will strengthen the behavior that worked.

3) *Antecedents*

The next variable in the learning equation is the immediate antecedent. Broadly speaking, an antecedent is whatever changes in the environment the moment before a behavior occurs. For example, in our introduction, we met Jamaal, who makes odd faces and adopts unusual postures whenever other children try to interact with him. In this example, what the peer says or does is the immediate antecedent to the behavior.

There are different types of antecedents that are important in functional behavior assessment. The first type of antecedent acts as a cue that reinforcement is available for performing a certain behavior. For example, an "open" sign on the door of Dunkin Donuts acts as a cue that coffee is available if you order and pay for it. For someone deprived of coffee (an EO is in effect), the open sign on the door provides a cue that reinforcement is available for coffee-purchasing behaviors. Similarly, for a child deprived of social praise (an EO for praise is in effect), the appearance of someone who has provided social praise in the past provides a cue that reinforcement is available for behaving in ways that have elicited praise before. This person's appearance on the scene acts as a big "open" sign on a Dunkin Donuts' door might. The technical name for these types of antecedents, which prompt someone to engage in a behavior in order to receive reinforcement, is a "discriminative stimulus" or "S^D".

Another type of antecedent that is important in understanding challenging behavior is one that has been associated with punishment for a certain behavior in the past. For example,

Dad walking into the room might be this kind of antecedent for a teenager who is smoking. Dad's appearance may cue him to hide his cigarettes if he has learned that smoking in his father's presence will result in punishment (even though more desirable consequences may be available for this behavior in the presence of his friends). This special type of antecedent is called a "punishing stimulus" or "S^P". The presence of S^D's and S^P's in an individual's world help determine whether or not he will perform a certain behavior at a given time.

Finally, there are novel or neutral antecedents. These are events that may have never occurred in the past or may not have been paired with consequences significant to you in the past. Some of these events will elicit behavior because you associate them with other, similar events. For example, if an insect that you have never seen before lands on your arm, you might swat it because of its association with mosquitoes or bees landing on your arm—an event that may have been paired with aversive consequences in the past. Other unfamiliar events may elicit novel responses from you as you attempt to respond effectively to them. For example, if you buy a new water toy for your child, you may try an extensive repertoire of actions, attempting to fill it up, before you stumble on the behavior that leads you to reinforcement (succeeding in filling the toy as you were motivated to do). In the future, that toy will serve as an S^D for the filling response that worked. In sum, learning is constant and ongoing and these novel or neutral antecedents are an essential part of this process.

Keep It Simple Summary

Antecedents are events that occur just before a behavior. There are three types:
1. an antecedent that cues an individual that a certain behavior will be reinforced (S^D);
2. an antecedent that cues an individual that a certain behavior will be punished (S^P);
3. a novel or neutral antecedent that leads to ongoing learning.

4) Behavior

The final variable critical to learning is behavior. A behavior is whatever an individual is doing. Examples include: smoking, making faces and postures, or head banging. Those are problematic behaviors that we want to decrease. However, there are also an infinite number of adaptive or helpful behaviors, such as talking to friends, looking at a speaker, completing homework, washing hands, walking, etc. These are behaviors that we want to increase. While there are some behaviors that are not observable, such as statements that you make silently to yourself (e.g., "Uh-oh, I can't remember that woman's name—is it Joan? Jada? Jill? Oh no, she's coming over here!"), this book will focus on public and observable behaviors only. For more information on unobservable, private events, see B. F. Skinner's (1953) book, *Science and Human Behavior,* or his (1984) article on the subject, "The Operational Analysis of Psychological Terms."

When designing an intervention for a problem behavior based on learning, we will consider all types of behaviors, rather than just challenging behaviors. Just as hitting your brother is termed a "behavior," handing your brother a cupcake is also called a "behavior." For every behavior that we will attempt to decrease using functional assessment, we will also identify at least one other behavior that we'd like to see more of. To complete a functional assessment, we will need information on an individual's skills as well as his deficits. As we will see in the next section of the book, when intervening with challenging behaviors, we have to be very precise in our thinking about behaviors. As part of a functional assessment we will develop careful definitions of specific behaviors and ensure that we define our target behaviors using measurable and reliable terms.

Keep It Simple Summary

A behavior is anything that a person does.

Putting the Four Learning Variables Together

In order for learning to occur, all four variables must be in place. For example, consider a child, Jessica, who is learning to ask for juice.

If the EO for juice is absent (let's say she just drank two big glasses of juice), then she will not make a juice request, and juice would not act as a reinforcer. Likewise, if Jessica has learned that Mommy cues the availability of juice and Mommy is not in the room, no juice request will occur. If Jessica has an EO for juice, and Mommy comes in the room, but Jessica is involved with a toy and, by the time she looks for Mommy to request the juice, Mommy is already gone, then the behavior of requesting juice will not be strengthened. Finally, if Jessica has an EO for juice, and she sees Mommy, and she requests juice, and Mommy tells her she cannot have juice right now, then requesting juice will be less likely in the future.

Considering all four variables allows us to create the following equations:

Motivation + Antecedent + Behavior + Consequence = Learning

EO + S^D + Behavior + Reinforcement = Learning

**Deprivation of juice for a given length of time +
the presence of Mommy + requesting juice + delivery of juice =
Increased likelihood of requesting juice in the future**

Keeping in mind that the above assumes that juice is not available without the request, learning has taken place. In the future, under similar conditions (the EO is in effect and the S^D is present), the behaviors are likely to recur.

Learning Theory and Problem Behaviors: The Functions of Behavior

Learning theory explains how people develop particular behaviors. Just as people learn useful behaviors, such as buying coffee or brushing their teeth, they also learn maladaptive behaviors, such as aggression or stereotypic behavior. When we do a functional assessment, we are actually trying to analyze how a behavior was learned. In this way, we can discover how to help someone "un-learn" it, and instead learn a new way to get his needs met. Earlier, a "function" of a behavior was described as the purpose it serves for the individual. Within the context of learning theory, we can offer a more specific discussion of what the term "function" involves.

Understanding a function of a behavior primarily involves a relationship between the EO and the reinforcer. An individual is deprived of something (creating an EO) and is therefore motivated to obtain it (the reinforcer). By analyzing this motivation and rein-forcement pairing, we can determine the function of a behavior. In the example described above in which Anthony hits his head and obtains beads, the function of the behavior is to obtain the beads. In the example described above in which Grace assaults her peers, the function of the behavior is to obtain peer attention.

The function of the behavior is the "payoff"—the reason for the behavior. The function of the behavior is the message that it com-municates: "I want beads" or "I want your attention," for example. Surprisingly, there are a very limited number of messages that a problem behavior communicates. While different professionals characterize these possible functions in slightly different ways, these different systems are equivalent to one another (e.g., Iwata, et al, 1982; Durand & Crimmins, 1988). This book will characterize the possible functions of behavior into four groups:

1. Attention,
2. Objects and activities,
3. Escape/avoid,
4. Automatic reinforcement.

Each of the possible functions is discussed in detail below.

1) Attention

The first possible function of a behavior is to obtain attention. The attention can be of varying qualities. It can involve physical attention such as touching, hugging, or handholding. It can involve vocal attention such as loud, intense reactions, or quieter, milder reactions. It can involve visual attention such as certain facial expressions or more or less animated reactions. Sometimes the function of a behavior is to prevent divided attention or to obtain attention from a group of individuals. Alternatively, a behavior can function to obtain the attention of one specific individual.

When completing a functional behavior assessment, it is important to consider the specificity of the types of attention that an individual can be motivated to obtain. Otherwise, assessment results can be deceptive. For example, consider a child being cared for by a babysitter while his mother works in her home office. Behavior problems may occur even when he is receiving a rich level of attention from the babysitter. An onlooker might ask, "How can there be an EO for attention when he is receiving so much attention?" Nevertheless, if the child has reached his threshold of deprivation of his mother's attention specifically, and has learned that certain behaviors will cause her to stop her work and intervene, then the function of his behavior might be to get his mother's attention. Similarly, the function of challenging behaviors may be to obtain high intensity attention. An adult may be providing attention that is not very animated or excited, but a certain challenging behavior may bring about a very intense quality of attention.

Sometimes challenging behaviors appear to be spiteful or intentionally aimed at upsetting someone. For example, I have heard about smaller behaviors that were viewed in this way, such as when a teacher complains about a student who taps his desk all day, making a thoroughly irritating noise. I have also seen more complex behaviors viewed in this way, such as when a child destroys a sibling's art project after that sibling refuses to play with him. Even though the sibling may not be present at the moment the art project is destroyed, a certain quality of attention is inevitable later. Similarly, adults may perceive some behaviors as "power struggles." These behaviors may be maintained by a certain, intense quality of attention.

As can be seen from the above examples, sometimes children are motivated to obtain attention that doesn't seem desirable to most people. While getting yelled at or moving a sibling to tears might not sound appealing to most, to some children, especially those with social disabilities, this consequence might be pretty attractive. Consider that these types of consequences are relatively predictable, intense, and require little effort to elicit, and the appeal becomes clearer. Furthermore, some children may not have the social skills to distinguish between desirable and undesirable social responses. Therefore, intense laughing and intense yelling may not appear that different.

The following is a list of ten common messages that an attention-maintained behavior may be communicating:

1. I want adult attention.
2. I want a particular adult's attention.
3. I want peer attention.
4. I want a particular peer's attention.
5. I want some physical contact.
6. I want a particular form of physical contact.
7. I want an intense emotional response.
8. I want a specific emotional response.
9. I want you all to myself.
10. I want a particular social interaction (e.g., a walk through the hall to "calm down," a deep massage from the OT, etc.).

2) Objects and Activities

Some children engage in problem behaviors as a means of gaining access to preferred objects or activities. This may seem confusing at first. For a child to learn a behavior with this function, he would have to be rewarded with something preferred after he engages in the problem behavior. You might question who would ever do this. When does a child misbehave and then get handed his favorite toy? While this may sound like an unlikely scenario, it actually happens quite often. For example, think about the typically developing child who has learned that if he throws a tantrum in the checkout aisle of the grocery store, his mother or father will buy him a candy bar to get him to stop making such a scene.

Where children with autism are concerned, parents and teachers often use access to object or activities as part of their intervention strategies for managing behavior. Consider Anthony and his beads. It is not at all uncommon for parents and teachers to use distraction or redirection to stop a difficult behavior. Another familiar strategy is to provide calming props, such as stress balls, silly putty, Koosh balls, etc., only when the child engages in challenging behaviors. This may result in a pattern similar to what we saw with Anthony: "I have no putty—I engage in a problem behavior—I have putty." Using various occupational therapy techniques after a challenging behavior (e.g., brushing, deep pressure, or swinging) may also trigger this pattern.

3) Escape/Avoid

As noted above, the most common function of challenging behaviors seen in school settings is escape. Certainly, school is rife with academic demands that a student may be motivated to escape from or avoid. However, children may also use problem behaviors to escape or avoid social demands. For some children, particularly those with autism spectrum disorders, social demands may be perceived as even more challenging than academic demands.

Behavioral researchers William Frea and Carolyn Hughes (1997) completed a functional assessment of inappropriate social behaviors, such as lack of eye contact or exaggerated emotional responses, made by adolescents with developmental disabilities. They found that escape from social interactions served as one function for these behaviors, which had previously been perceived as skill deficits. Jamaal's postures and facial expressions, described in the Introduction, may illustrate this function. Recall that he demonstrated appropriate interaction skills with adults, exhibited these odd-looking behaviors only when approached by peers, and the behaviors resulted in the peers ceasing to interact with him.

Finally, someone might also exhibit a certain behavior to escape or avoid a certain type of stimulation. Consider the unusual sensitivities experienced by many children with autism spectrum disorders. Lights, sounds, and textures that are innocuous to parents and teachers may be extremely distressful to these children. One preschooler I worked with had severe tantrums every time she had to get on her bus home. Finally, after some frustrating guess work, the team decided just to ask her what she didn't like about the bus. She explained that the checkered pattern on the seats hurt her ears. It would have been impossible for any of the team members to predict that looking at a certain pattern would hurt a student's ears. We switched her bus to one with a different pattern on the seats and the tantrums disappeared.

The following is a list of ten common messages that an escape-maintained behavior may be communicating:

1. I don't want to do this work—it's too hard, easy, uninteresting to me, or non-functional.
2. I don't want to talk to you, or you to talk to me.
3. I don't want you to touch me.
4. I don't want to play this.
5. I don't know how or don't want to manage this unstructured time. This is a very challenging demand for me.
6. I don't want to be around this visual input.
7. I don't want to be around these sounds.
8. I don't want to be around this smell.
9. I don't want to touch this texture.
10. I don't want to eat this food.

4) Automatic Reinforcement

Some behaviors occur in response to internal antecedents and consequences. These behaviors satisfy a need for some type of internal stimulation rather than the more common external motivators. Because the antecedents and consequences for these behaviors cannot be observed, this function (automatic reinforcement) is proposed when no environmental changes are noted before or after the behavior occurs.

While any behavior can serve any function, and one cannot tell the function of the behavior by looking at it, some examples of behaviors that might illustrate this function could include: talking to oneself (the sound of one's voice is reinforcing), watching one's fingers (the visual stimulation is reinforcing), or rocking (the kinesthetic feedback is reinforcing). Hallmarks of this type of behavior are that it can occur when someone is alone or in a very non-stimulating environment, but not necessarily. It can occur any place or time where the self-stimulatory behavior is more reinforcing than whatever is going on outside of the individual's skin. Automatically reinforced behaviors are also common when an individual is experiencing some pain (e.g., biting objects when experiencing a toothache, or banging the side of one's head or pulling one's ears when experiencing an earache). For this reason, if an automatically reinforcing behavior involving the body suddenly crops up in someone who might not have the skills to report some pain or discomfort, it might pay to have a quick evaluation from a relevant medical professional.

In terms of a functional assessment, compulsive behaviors, such as those associated with Obsessive Compulsive Disorder, occur in response to internal cues and are subsequently reinforced by some type of internal stimulation. These, too would be identified as automatically reinforcing. Similarly, it can be challenging to distinguish tics from a learned automatic reinforcement behavior, or a learned behavior with some other function. If you do come across a behavior that is difficult to differentiate from another behavioral diagnosis and it turns out to serve an automatic reinforcement function, you may want to consult with a professional who has expertise in the disorder the behavior resembles. Traditional medical or behavioral treatments for other disorders may be effective in individuals with an additional autism spectrum disorder.

While stereotypy (repetitive, non-purposeful behavior) is often assumed to always be automatically reinforced, this is not an accurate assumption. Stereotypy can serve any function. One school-aged child I worked with who had autism and was also blind provides a clear illustration of how tricky identifying the function of stereotypy can be. During the winter, when the ground was icy, Samantha would jump up and down and flap her hands each day when she got off her school bus. This terrified her mother, who feared that her daughter would injure herself on the ice. Although I began the functional assessment with as open a mind as possible, I had to fight my assumption that jumping and flapping was automatically reinforced. My first clue that something else was going on occurred when Samantha's father mentioned that when he took her off the bus, rather than her mother, the behaviors did not occur.

Further assessment revealed that Samantha's mother responded to the jumping and flapping by putting her arm around Samantha and walking her into the house, which her father did not do. As Samantha had to use her cane to find her way into the house without this assistance and this was a new and challenging skill for her, her mother's guidance made the walk into the house significantly easier for her. To assess the hypothesis that she jumped and flapped to obtain this assistance from her mother, we tried having her mother watch her from the window instead of meeting her at the bus. Samantha immediately stopped jumping and flapping. The S^D signaling reinforcement for this behavior (i.e., her mother waiting at the bus stop) was no longer present. As her mother switched to this routine permanently, the behavior disappeared.

5) Behaviors That Serve More Than One Function

Some behaviors serve more than one function at a time. For example, making a wisecrack in class might result in being sent to the principal's office (escaping a task) and might also make the rest of the students laugh (accessing peer attention). In this example, one behavior serves two functions at the same time. The same student might make a wisecrack when there is no work demand in order to get peer attention or when he is alone with his teacher in order to escape work. In this case, the behavior serves one function at one time and another function later.

Furthermore, a behavior can serve three functions or all four functions. For example, imagine an adolescent who smears his feces. This behavior may begin as a function of automatic reinforcement: perhaps he was uncomfortable with the feces in his pants and attempts to remove it with his hands. He then wipes his hands off on a nearby object. However, he soon discovers that this makes the staff members at his job site, a 7-11 convenience store, move away from him immediately. He has now learned that smearing feces is an effective means of escaping interactions with these unfamiliar adults. Furthermore, the staff at 7-11 inevitably report this behavior to the job coach. A lengthy interaction with the familiar and preferred job coach may ensue as he scrubs the feces with a particular scrub brush that he enjoys using. The behavior has now been further strengthened by both attention and access to preferred objects. A behavior as powerful as this might even generalize to the next setting, as, if it persists, he is likely to be fired from his current position.

If an individual is using challenging behaviors to communicate multiple functions, this is a cue to the parent or teacher that there is some communication problem. Either the individual needs to develop a more efficient means of communicating basic needs, or, for whatever reason, appropriate communication is not being sufficiently reinforced.

It is also important to note that more than one behavior can be used to serve the same function. A child may have a broad repertoire of behaviors to choose from in getting a certain need met. For example, to escape work, a student might sometimes make wisecracks, sometimes rip up his assignments, and sometimes destroy school property. In this case, the student has many means of communicating the same message. In the next section, we will explore how someone determines which behavior he will demonstrate at which time.

How Does My Child Choose a Behavior to Use?

As noted above, a child may have many inappropriate behaviors that all serve the same function. Furthermore, he may have many appropriate behaviors that serve the same function as the inappropriate behavior. For example, let's say that a child's mother is on the phone and he wants her attention. He might say, "Excuse

A Special Note on Choice and Control

Clients I have worked with often wonder about the value of control. Do our children sometimes try out a challenging behavior just to have a little power or to assert their right to make choices? I have found that interventions based on the four functions described above are successful without the addition of this "fifth function." Nevertheless, we have probably all seen behaviors that are hard to think of another way.

As a matter of good behavioral "hygiene," to prevent behavior problems, always ensure that your child has plenty of opportunities to direct his own destiny throughout the day. You may be surprised at how many opportunities to make choices you can offer. For example, your child may not be able to choose whether or not to get dressed for the day, but he may be able to choose whether to brush his teeth or put on his clothes first, which shoes to wear, and where to put them on.

me," he might just start telling her something that happened, he might tell her he needs her to take him to the bathroom, he might pull his baby sister's hair, or he might pour soda on the living room floor. Each of these behaviors has some probability of getting his mother's attention. For most behaviors in a person's repertoire, both appropriate and inappropriate, there are usually many options of behaviors an individual might choose to meet his needs.

Given that many behaviors can serve the same function, how does an individual select which behavior to perform? One answer lies in the efficiency of the behavior. First of all, efficiency is evaluated in terms of how much effort is required to perform the behavior. For example, the young girl with autism who was also blind (described above) figured out that it was easier for her to flap her hands, jump, and be guided up the walk by her mother than it was for her to use her cane.

To encourage an individual to select an appropriate behavior, we have to ensure that he is proficient enough at performing this behavior and that it is not hard work for him. Some people's inappropriate behaviors can be treated by having them practice a simple and appropriate alternative until they can perform it effortlessly. The young man described above who was given a picture card to request his cushiony restraint provides an example of this approach.

Next, an individual is more likely to select a behavior that is likely to produce the greatest amount of reinforcement. For example, if raising your hand in class leads to a neutral, "Yes, Johnny," but throwing pencils leads to a very intense, one-to-one discussion in the hallway, a student with an EO for intense attention is likely to request it by throwing pencils. Similarly, whichever behavior gets the reinforcer the fastest gets priority. If Johnny raises his hand and has to wait three minutes to be called on, or he calls out and gets attention right away, the behavioral pendulum will swing in favor of calling out.

Finally, all of these variables are considered together. The behavior that is ultimately selected represents a balance of:

1. effort required to obtain the reinforcer,
2. quantity of the reinforcer provided, and
3. immediacy of the reinforcer.

Traditionally held beliefs about why behavior occurs all fall someplace within the model described in this chapter. For example, the function of almost every behavior you can think of can be boiled down to either a desire for attention, escape, a particular object or activity, or automatic reinforcement. For instance, on the surface, students who behave well in class may be assumed to be doing so to please the teacher. However, the function of pleasing another person is a subset of obtaining (positive) attention. Or, for another example, in everyday life it is common to attribute someone's behavior to being in a "bad mood." In fact, an individual's mood can change his threshold for motivation to engage in a behavior, but expressing that mood does not actually serve as a function of behavior. (Think of a child with autism who is able to tell his brother "Go away" when he is feeling relatively calm in his own home, but who bites other people to get them to go away when he is in frightening, unfamiliar environment.) Deciding whether or not to do the "right" thing will also always require a calculation of the balance of effort and reinforcement.

Some behaviors occur due to a pattern related to what has been learned in the past rather than as a result of immediate reinforcement. For example, reinforcing a two-year-old for sharing, helping others, and being gentle strengthens a broader "response class" (group of related behaviors) that can be referred to as altruism or caring for others. Later, as an adult, this former two-year-old might share food with the poor or rescue someone from a shark as a result of this strong response class, rather than to obtain a specific reinforcer at that moment. In other words, behaviors may be learned according to one of the four functions of behaviors that are maintained on only a weak or intermittent schedule.

3 | Getting Started
First Steps for Completing a Functional Behavior Assessment

You've mastered the basic concepts of the learning process. Now you're ready to use what you've learned to complete a functional behavior assessment. The next five chapters will cover the assessment process in a step-by-step fashion. These chapters are designed to be a practical guide and are therefore geared towards organization and efficiency. Tips to keep things simple will be offered. The following topics will be covered:

Step 1: Create an assessment team.
Step 2: Select a target behavior.
Step 3: Define the target behavior.
Step 4: Measure the target behavior.
Step 5: Establish a baseline.
Step 6: Interview team members.
Step 7: Observe the behavior.
Step 8: Experiment with the behavior.

Step 1: Create an Assessment Team

Once you have decided to address a particular behavior, the first step is to identify appropriate team members. Careful attention should be paid to this part of the assessment process, as one person's information can be the key to solving the mystery of a problem behavior.

Consider the example in Chapter 2 involving Samantha, the girl with autism who was also blind. My consultation visits with the family took place at a day and time when her father was usually at work. Because Samantha's mother was the primary caregiver, I didn't think that this would be a problem. Nevertheless, I happened to come a different day one week and met with her father. It was his information that ultimately led to identifying the correct function of the behavior.

Ideally, anyone who has seen the targeted behavior should participate on the assessment team, at least in the information gathering process. Additionally, anyone who is knowledgeable about the child's patterns of skills and deficits, particularly related to communication, should participate as well. Even if an individual has not seen the behavior firsthand, he or she may be able to contribute information about variables in place and the skills being practiced when the behavior does *not* occur.

Family Members

Usually, the team begins with the child's family. Although parents play the most pivotal roles on an assessment team, even a preschool-aged sibling might be able to offer insights about what is likely to set off or prevent a behavior. It is surprising what good behaviorists young children can be! Probably out of necessity, they are often very skilled in recognizing cues that a problem behavior is coming. Some siblings can easily prevent or escape a problem behavior, while others might actually have some experience intentionally provoking the problem behavior. Anyone with an older brother or sister who has been a victim of silent poking, prodding, or pinching, only to get in trouble for the louder and more public retaliation, recognizes this ability in siblings.

Professionals

Professionals who support the family in meeting their child's needs should also participate on the assessment team. This might include the child's teacher, speech therapist, occupational therapist, or home programmer, among others. These individuals may each have different observations and experiences with the problem behavior. Furthermore, each may have different insights into the child's pattern of skills and deficits that has made the problem behavior the most efficient choice for her in getting what she needs.

The assessment process suffers when people who might be aware of variables affecting the problem behavior are excluded. To prevent this from happening on your assessment team, try to think out of the box. Include everyone who might have helpful information. Would your child's bus driver possibly have seen the problem behavior? Are the "specials" teachers (e.g., Art, Music, Physical Education) included in the team meeting? Would your child's grandparents have valuable input? How about the lunch aide? Or the playground monitor? Be sure to consider all possible contributors. Also, try to allow each observer to speak for him- or herself. If you allow one person to summarize the thoughts of another, you risk losing something critical in the translation.

Peers

Peers are an often overlooked, but potentially valuable source of information about children in regular education settings. Like siblings, peers may be very skilled at recognizing what sets off a problem behavior and knowing how to prevent it. Nevertheless, approaching a peer for information requires keen sensitivity to the confidentiality needs of the child with ASD. If a peer witnesses a problem behavior, it is relatively easy for educational staff to say, "What happened over here?" as they would with any other student.

However, in investigating an ongoing problem behavior that hasn't just occurred, questioning a peer requires more judgment. A first consideration is whether or not peers are aware that a given child has special needs. If peers are aware of their classmate's special needs, then approach peers casually without drawing any undue attention to the student. You might say something like, "I've noticed that you boys usually play on the same equipment as Johnny does on the playground. I've also noticed that he often bites his hand when he is playing there. He really likes that equipment, so I hate to keep him from it, but I don't want him to hurt himself. Do you boys have any ideas about what might set him off there? Or do you have any ideas about how to prevent him from biting his hand?" You might be surprised by the insightfulness of their responses. You can also use this kind of approach to address problems in the peers' own behavior (e.g., "How can we help you stay in your seat until the end of lunch?") so that these types of conversations about a student with special needs won't stand out.

Sometimes peers are not aware that a child has any special needs. In this situation, team members must either seek parents' permission to share this information, or prioritize preserving the child's confidentiality. One strategy some teachers use to gather information without sacrificing confidentiality is to solicit ideas during a group discussion about problem behaviors in the class more generally. In the midst of exploring factors leading to calling out, teasing, etc., the target behavior can be discussed.

Another strategy teachers might use is to distribute question-naires to the class, asking the students to identify a problematic be-havior that they observed another child perform, and then answer questions about it. For example, you might ask the class to: "Name a behavior that you have seen at school which causes a problem for the student performing the behavior or for those around him or her. Answer the following questions with that behavior in mind." You can then progress to asking what typically happens before or after the behavior, and other assessment-based questions posed at an age appropriate level. Responses can then be used as part of a broader discussion of citizenship, but peer observations about the problem behavior are now available. This strategy will only work if the problem behavior is dramatic enough that a significant number of peers are likely to choose that as their target behavior.

The Child

A final critical source of information that is also often over-looked is the child herself. Recall the preschooler who shared that the checkered pattern on the bus seats hurt her ears. Information this specific would never have been available through an observer. When working with a verbal child, simply asking a few questions about why the behavior occurs or when it is hardest to resist sometimes provides tremendous insight and should be a routine part of the assessment process. In fact, students as young as fifth through eighth grade have successfully completed extensive assessment interviews geared toward identifying the causes of their own problem behaviors with results that were similar to those of their teachers (Reed, Thomas, Sprague & Horner, 1997). An alternative functional assessment interview has been used with elementary school children, but preliminary investigation seems to suggest that the age of the responder may influence the interview's usefulness (Kern, Dunlap, Clarke, & Childs, 1994). Examples of assessment interviews are on pages 67-72 and 80-81.

Assigning Roles to Team Members

Each team member will have a specific role in the functional behavior assessment process. The team leader or coordinator has the most central role. This person's job description includes arranging communication among team members, overseeing the implementation of assessment procedures, and making decisions about how data will be collected and analyzed. This person needs strong organizational skills as well as a solid understanding of functional behavior assessment. Typically, this role would fall to a parent, a teacher, or a behavior specialist helping with the behavior.

Next, some team members will act as informants. They will answer interview questions, take data as assigned to them by the coordinator, and report any observations or ideas. These are great roles for siblings, grandparents, specials teachers, etc. Finally, some team members may assist the team leader in analyzing and interpreting the data. This might be a behavior specialist helping a teacher (or vice versa), a teacher helping a parent (or vice versa), etc. Roles should be assigned based on interest, commitment, and expertise, rather than on title.

Keep It Simple Summary

Take information from whomever you can! Be sure that the assessment team has a leader to coordinate and organize team members and information. And don't forget to get information from the individual with autism whenever possible too!

Step 2: Select a Target Behavior

Many children with autism spectrum disorders have more than one problematic behavior. Deciding how or where to start in improving behavior often poses a challenge. The guidelines that follow will help the team focus and prioritize in order to make their to-do list a manageable one.

Guideline 1: Address Only One Behavior at a Time

If at all possible, focus on just one behavior at a time. As we proceed in describing the assessment process, you will see that treating each behavior requires observation, data collection, and, ultimately, a plan to address it. In other words, tackling each behavior problem involves a significant amount of work. Targeting more than one behavior at a time may overwhelm team members. This may lead them to cut corners in their data collection, observe less closely, or feel hopeless in achieving their goals. As a result, this may slow down the successful assessment for all behaviors. Instead, to the extent possible, limit the demands on team members, consequently setting them up for success in the assessment process.

Additionally, remember that people with autism spectrum disorders often have more than one behavior that serves a particular function. Assessment results for one behavior could lead to an intervention that addresses all behaviors with this function. An intervention plan based on a functional behavior assessment of one behavior often affects other behaviors as well. After addressing the first behavior, the other behaviors may no longer require intervention. For example, let's revisit our wisecracking, homework- ripping, property-destroying student who is motivated to escape his work. A functional assessment of wisecracking alone would lead to an intervention geared toward escape from work—perhaps the work would be peppered with topics he enjoys and he would be allowed to request breaks each day by raising his hand and asking appropriately. This would not only decrease wisecracking, but would also decrease any other behavior serving an escape function.

Guideline 2: Habilitation

A general guideline that behavior analysts use when decid-ing what to teach is referred to as *habilitation*. This means that you develop goals designed to increase someone's access to naturally occurring, unplanned reinforcement and minimize her access to naturally occurring, unplanned punishment. For example, if Gary, a young child with Asperger's disorder, desperately wants to make friends, but the other children avoid him because he spends a lot of time talking about fonts, then intervention might start by decreasing font-talk around peers. This would increase Gary's opportunities to get positive feedback from peers. Similarly, if an adolescent girl gets kicked off of a city bus for sitting too close to people, and she needs the bus to get to the after-school job that she loves, then the first behavior to assess would be sitting too close to people. This would ensure that she keeps her job, through which she receives reinforcement.

According to the principle of habilitation, behavior problems that interfere with adaptive functioning for the individual or mem-bers of her community must be addressed right away. Examples might include behaviors that prevent a student from completing her work in school, that prevent peers on a sports team from hear-ing the coach's instruction, or that prevent a child from taking care of her hygiene at home.

Be careful to avoid addressing behaviors simply because they annoy you. This violates the principle of habilitation. For example, if a student hums quietly while completing written tasks, and only does this with her one-to-one instructor, there is no reason to address this behavior. If she can still learn and will not be handicapped by this behavior in any way, then there is no impact on her access to reinforcement or punishment. If she wants to hum quietly for these tasks, it is her right to choose to do so. Since I've never met a parent or teacher with too much time or energy on their hands, it would be a shame to waste precious resources on a problem that will not change the individual's life in any way. It would certainly be easier for the instructor to learn to tolerate his student's humming.

In contrast, let's imagine that the student above hummed in her inclusive classroom, on the bus, and at the mall. Let's further imagine that her peers made fun of her for this and refused to sit near her in school. This would be an example where the same behavior was leading to naturally occurring punishers, which may unfortunately not be strong enough to stop the behavior on their own. In this case, a functional assessment-based intervention would be warranted.

Guideline 3: Be Safe

Always address behaviors that pose a danger to self, others, or property before addressing less threatening concerns. Preserving the safety of the person with ASD and those around him or her takes precedence over everything else.

Usually, you will complete a functional behavior assessment on a dangerous behavior as you would with any other behavior. However, some behaviors are so dangerous that something must be done immediately as a stopgap and the assessment must wait. In this case, you would be using a crisis management approach.

The basic principle behind crisis management is finding strategies to avoid the behavior or minimize its impact in the moment that it occurs rather than making any long-term improvement in the behavior. Unfortunately, this might even mean that you need to reinforce a problem behavior. Once everyone is safe, a more thorough and long-term approach can be identified. For example, if a student is throwing objects at classmates to escape a task, remove the task immediately to preserve the other children's safety, even though this reinforces the problem behavior. After everyone is safe, then you can begin to think of an assessment plan. Crisis management is discussed again in Chapter 9.

Guideline 4: Set the Child and the Assessment Team Up for Success

If the above guidelines leave you with multiple options of behaviors to address, tackle the simplest problem behavior first. This will allow the child and the intervention team to experience success, which in turn is likely to breed more success in the future. Typically, the newest behavior or the behavior that occurs in the fewest settings will be the easiest to assess and ultimately treat. Similarly, if a problem behavior seems fairly straightforward as you think about why it might be occurring, that behavior might be a good choice for a starting point.

Guideline 5: Consider the Needs of Significant Others

In combination with the above guidelines, consider the needs of significant others when selecting a target behavior. For example, there may be time constraints on a family that make assessment of a particular behavior urgent. Perhaps a child has a behavior problem that occurs in crowds and her older sister is getting married in three months. This behavior would need to be targeted immediately. Alternatively, a problem behavior may restrict a family's participation in valued activities (e.g., attending church services or going to concerts). Then this behavior becomes a priority. Finally, some challenging behaviors make everyday life difficult for family members. One teenaged sibling that I met with had a brother who stripped in public. She was terrifically embarrassed to ever leave the house with her family and avoided it at all costs. Behaviors with such a strong impact on others cry out for immediate attention.

Practice Examples

Let's do a couple of quick practice examples in selecting a behavior to target:

Joe

Joe is a twelve-year-old boy with PDD-NOS and mental retardation who is included in a regular education classroom. Joe has been included for three years and has formed wonderful relationships with his peers, which he deeply values. This year, Joe is exhibiting more problem behaviors than he has in the past. Specifically, he makes a clicking sound with his mouth, which most people do not notice, but his teachers, who know him very well, can detect. Additionally, he is laughing loudly and inappropriately during class. When he does this his teachers give him a stern look, which prompts Joe to engage in a lengthy discussion with them about whether or not they are mad at him. Finally, Joe has started biting others. To date, he has bitten two peers and a teacher. Where should we start with Joe?

The first behavior to address with Joe is the biting. This is a dangerous behavior and therefore takes priority. This is also a good place to start because if he continues to bite peers, his relationships with them may fall into jeopardy (minimizing his access to reinforcement). Additionally, the biting is a relatively new behavior and therefore will be the most likely to respond to assessment and intervention. Next, the team will target his non-contextual laughing. This distracts his peers and may interfere with their learning. It also interferes with Joe's learning, as it results in lengthy discussions with teachers that ultimately take time away from work. Finally, there is no reason to address the clicking sounds. They do not impede his progress in any way.

Tracy

Tracy is an adult with high functioning autism who lives in a supervised apartment. Tracy desperately wants a romantic relationship but has not yet found the right partner. In fact, she has not yet formed any peer friendships, which she also craves. While Tracy speaks easily about topics of interest to her with familiar caregivers, she will not respond to her peers' attempts to interact with her. During planned social groups, she is likely to engage in disruptive behaviors, such as breaking task materials, as well as aggressive behaviors, throwing materials at other people in the group.

The first behavior to address for Tracy is the aggression. As with Joe, dangerous behaviors take priority. Additionally, it is likely that only so many instances of aggression will be tolerated before she is asked to leave the social group. Because Tracy is so interested in forming relationships, the group is a critical potential source of reinforcement for her. Next, breaking task materials could be addressed for similar reasons. Finally, failure to respond to social initiations must be targeted. This behavior clearly thwarts Tracy's goals for herself and should be addressed through the functional assessment process rather than chalking it up to a skills deficit or anxiety.

Keep It Simple Summary

Always address dangerous behaviors first. Next, consider behaviors that are impeding access to reinforcement or leading to undue punishment for the individual, her community members, or her significant others. All other things being equal, address the behavior that is most likely to lead to success first.

Step 3: Define the Target Behavior

Many parents and teachers are confused when I ask them to write a definition of the problem behavior. They might look at me in disbelief and ask, "You don't know what a tantrum is?" The problem is that what I call a tantrum might not be the same as what that parent calls a tantrum. The same is true for head banging, echoing, spitting, screaming, or any other problem behavior you can imagine. Because behaviors are assessed by a team of people who each need to know what the others mean by what they say, it is imperative that a clear definition of the behavior be developed.

The best way to write a definition of a behavior is to jot down instructions to someone else about how to act it out. Pretend you are a director giving instruction to an actor as to how to play the part of your child. Write down exactly what to do. This will lead to a clear definition of the behavior. For example, if I were defining my two-year-old son's tantrums, I would write something like: "Run to nearest couch, chair, or bed while yelling, "No!" and throw self onto the furniture belly first." Anyone reading this could probably act this out and look just like my son. To test whether or not your definition will be functional, write it out and give the definition to someone who has never seen your child's problem behavior. Ask him or her to act it out. If it looks right, then you have a clear definition.

Some problem behaviors are not exactly the same every time. For example, "oppositional behavior" might sometimes involve screaming, "No!", sometimes involve pretending not to hear what was asked, and sometimes involve saying, "Do it yourself!" When different behaviors tend to occur together or tend to follow the same antecedent, you can group them together with an "or" statement and then address them accordingly. For example, the operational definition for the oppositional behavior described above might be something like: "When given an instruction [child] either screams, 'No!', screams, 'Do it yourself!', or continues whatever he was doing."

Ultimately, you will use your definition to measure the behavior. Depending on what the behavior looks like, you will want to know how many times it occurred, how long it lasted, or how intense it was. Therefore, you must write your definition in a way that allows the behavior to be measured. To the extent possible, try to ensure that each definition clarifies the beginning and end of the problem behavior. It must be clear to the reader when to count a behavior as one long instance of the behavior, or when to start counting anew. If intensity is an issue, each intensity level must be clearly defined.

It is best to choose what to count (how many, how intense, or how long) before writing a definition to ensure compatibility between the definition and the measuring device. For example, you wouldn't want to count the duration of the tantrum with the definition of my son's tantrum above. When would you start timing—when he runs or when he throws himself on the couch? When would you stop timing—when he flops onto the couch or when he gets up from the couch? What if he is crying when he gets up from the couch? What if he runs directly to another couch? Is that a new episode to time or the same one? In contrast, that definition would be very easy to use when measuring the frequency of the behavior: each time he runs to a couch and flops on it while yelling is one tantrum. A full discussion of guidelines for deciding what to count will be presented Chapter 4.

Keep It Simple Summary

To create a definition of a problem behavior, write out instructions for someone to act it out. Actually give the instructions to someone who has never seen the behavior. If he or she acts it out correctly, you have a clear definition.

4 | Measuring Behavior

Once you have identified a problem behavior for intervention, defined it so that anyone can recognize it, and selected a team to help you understand the function of the behavior, you are ready for the next steps in FBA: deciding what parameters you will use to measure the behavior and then using those parameters to measure the behavior before you begin to intervene. Steps for completing both of these tasks are described below.

Step 4: Measure the Target Behavior

As part of our functional behavior assessment, we need to quantify the behavior. This allows us to compare the strength of the behavior in different contexts, to identify trends in the behavior, and to ultimately evaluate whether or not the plan that results from our functional assessment is working. Measurements of the behavior provide the facts upon which our functional behavior assessment is based. Without our data, we would just be guessing at the behavior's function. This section will describe practical strategies to get the measuring done. A blank data sheet for each type of measurement system is included so that you may copy it and use it when you are ready to complete your assessment.

In choosing how to measure a behavior, consider two questions:
1. What will be the easiest way to measure this behavior?
2. What measure will be the most likely to capture behavior change?

You want a measure that all team members can use reliably, as well as a measure that will help you see whether or not the intervention that you develop based on your assessment is working. Some behaviors have a more obvious start and finish than others and do not happen in quick succession with other instances of the behavior. For these behaviors, measuring frequency would be effective. Examples include my son's tantrum and Joe's bites described in Chapter 3, or the number of wisecracks made by our student who wants to escape his work. Other behaviors may not be as discrete. These incidents may involve the same behavior repeating itself in rapid succession (e.g., head-banging), multiple behaviors happening in rapid succession (e.g., an aggressive incident involving hitting, kicking, and biting), or may involve one or a number of behaviors that occur over a long period of time (e.g., crying with or without other tantrum-related behaviors). The best method of documenting improvement for these behaviors would probably be to measure the duration of the event.

Finally, progress in some behaviors can best be measured by changes in intensity. For example, a child who makes noise in synagogue might improve by getting quieter and quieter over time. A simple definition of levels of noise-making in synagogue that might work for this child could look like this:

- **Level One:** People in his row turn to see where the noise is coming from.
- **Level Two:** People in adjoining rows turn to see where the noise is coming from.
- **Level Three:** People in nearby rows turn to see where the noise is coming from.
- **Level Four:** People throughout the congregation turn to see where the noise is coming from.

It is easier to learn to define behaviors based on behaviors that you have actually seen. In order to practice using definitions of behaviors within the context of this book, below are two lists. On the left side of the page are behaviors that many people have seen in classic movies. On the right side of the page are their definitions. Try to match the behaviors with their definitions. In the list of answers, measurement strategies suited for each definition will be identified.

1. *Home Alone* Face	a) Toes touching with heels out forming a "V" with feet, pivot on toes to bring heels in to touch one another, and return to starting position repeatedly
2. Dorothy clicks her heels in the *Wizard of Oz*	b) Runs at victim, knocks him down on ground, punches victim's face repeatedly
3. Norman Bates stabbing his victim in the shower in *Psycho*	c) When holding ball for kicker, pulls ball away as kicker's foot is within 3 inches of making contact with ball
4. Ralphie beats up the bully in *A Christmas Story*	d) Hands on cheeks, mouth open wide, screaming
5. Lucy pulling the football away from Charlie Brown to make him fall	e) Grasping knife handle with one arm held straight over head, arm swings down to put knife in victim and repeat

Answers:
1. d) Use a measure of frequency or duration
2. a) Use a measure of duration
3. e) Use a measure of frequency
4. b) Use measure of intensity or duration (more definition needed for intensity)
5. c) Use a measure of frequency

Frequency Recording

Measuring frequency means that you are counting how many times something happens in a given period of time. You might record the number of times a behavior occurs per day. For instance, we could measure the number of comments Darra makes about Clay Aiken per day. You could also measure the number of occurrences of a behavior in an hour, a ten-minute sample of time, a semester, or any time period at all. It all depends on the nature of the behavior and the time constraints of the observer.

If you are observing for the same amount of time each observation, then you can simply jot down the total as your "data point" (record of performance for the day). However, if you are observing for a different period of time each day, then you'll need to calculate a rate. Rate is obtained by dividing the number of behaviors by the length of the observation period. For example, if a student rips his assignment page six times in the course of a six-hour school day, then he is ripping pages at a rate of one per hour (6 rips divided by 6 hours = 1 per hour). If a student calls out 10 times during a 20-minute observation, then he is calling out at a rate of 0.5 per minute (10 call outs divided by 20 minutes = 0.5 per minute).

Keep It Simple Summary

In order to make this type of data collection practical, consider the following tricks.

- Buy a golf counter, keep it in your pocket, and click it each time a behavior occurs. At the end of the observation period, you can look at the number on the counter to see how many times the behavior has occurred. This will keep your hands free during the day and prevent the need to carry a pen and paper or clipboard around with you. If you need to calculate a rate, be sure to jot down your start time and your end time.

- Wrap a piece of masking tape around your wrist and keep a marker in your pocket. You can make a mark on the tape each time the behavior occurs and then put the pen back in your pocket. At the end of the observation period, count up the hash marks on the tape to get your total. Again, this will prevent the need for a clipboard and keep your hands free. Remember to make note of your start time and end time if you need to calculate a rate.

- Keep pennies in your right pocket. Whenever the behavior occurs, transfer one penny to your left pocket. At the end of the observation, count up the pennies in your left pocket to get your total. You can do the same thing with objects in the area where you will be with your child. For example, if the behavior happens in the kitchen, pull one packet of sugar out of the sugar bowl each time the behavior occurs. Again, if you will be calculating a rate, you will need to record your start and end times.

- If carrying a clipboard with you will not interfere with your activity, then you can carry the Frequency Recording Data Sheet in Appendix A with you and simply make a hash mark for each occurrence of the behavior.

Measuring frequency or rate is ideal for very discrete behaviors with a clear beginning and end. This data is also very easy to collect because everyone has experience counting; you will not be asking any observers to do something new or unusual for them.

Time-Based Measures of Behavior

Duration

Measuring the duration of a behavior involves recording how long a behavior lasts. This type of measure is best suited for behaviors with a large number of component parts (e.g., a fist fight) or that last a long time (e.g., crying episodes). Some other examples of problem behaviors that might be conducive to a duration measure include rocking, tantrums, or off-task behavior. These behaviors may not include discrete episodes or may involve too many component parts of different types to measure. Note that when you measure duration, you automatically get a count of frequency. Each duration you record counts as one occurrence of the behavior.

To measure duration, you simply record the beginning and end time of the behavior and then figure out how long it lasted. You can measure duration in seconds, minutes, or hours. You can then calculate either an average or total duration per observation. A total duration is only appropriate for use when each observation lasts the same amount of time. Otherwise, the totals aren't comparable and an average will provide a better gauge.

You can measure duration of an *inappropriate* behavior during your assessment. This would imply that a longer duration involves more problematic behavior. Alternatively, you can measure duration of *appropriate* behavior during your assessment. Then a longer duration would imply less problematic behavior. For example, for a child who exhibits a variety of problematic, off-task behaviors during math lessons, it will be easier to measure the duration of on-task behavior during this time than to define each possible off-task behavior and measure each one. To measure on-task behavior, you would record the start and end time of each bout of on-task behavior and then calculate a total or average duration.

Keep It Simple Summary

In order to make this type of data collection practical, consider the following tricks.

- Use a timer that counts up. You can keep it in your pocket and just hit the start and stop buttons at the appropriate time. Keep a paper and pen in a nearby location and then jot down the durations. If you are calculating a total duration, you do not need to write anything until the end of the day or session. The timer will continue to add the durations for you.

- If you are in a room with a clock, look up and remember the start time. When the behavior ends, jot down both the start and end times. To do this, you can either carry a clipboard or keep a pen and paper in an accessible place.

- Buy a cheap watch with a big face and an eyeliner pencil. Keep the eyeliner pencil in your pocket. Mark the watch at the place where the minute hand is when the behavior starts and then again when the behavior stops. This will buy you a little time before you need to get to your data sheet. If you use this approach, be sure to jot the duration down as soon as possible after the behavior ends. If the marks from one occurrence are still on the watch when the next occurrence begins, it will be too confusing to determine which marks are from which behavior. Also, this may become confusing for behaviors that last more than an hour, as it will be unclear which is the start mark and which is the end mark. Wipe the watch face with a baby wipe after recording times on your data sheet.

- Use the Duration of Behavior or Latency to Behavior Data Sheets in Appendix B and Appendix C if you can carry a clipboard and pencil while observing the behavior.

Latency

Another time-based measure is the latency to a behavior. This refers to the amount of time that elapses between the onset of an event and the start of a behavior. Examples of latency measures include the length of time it takes you to get up after an alarm rings, the length of time it takes a child to begin working after instructions have been given, or the length of time a student participates in group before a problematic behavior occurs. Like duration, latency can be measured in seconds, minutes, or hours. To measure latency, you record the time that a stimulus is introduced or an activity begins (e.g., home-based discrete trial session starts), and then record the time that a behavior occurs (e.g., the child throws materials on floor). The amount of time that passes between the two events is the latency.

As with duration measures, either an appropriate or inappropriate behavior can be measured. For example, a longer latency to a problem behavior indicates improvement (e.g., more and more time passes before disruptive behavior in groups), or a shorter latency to an appropriate behavior can indicate improvement (e.g., less and less time passes before coming to group when called). Note that when you measure latency, you automatically get a count of frequency. Each latency that you record counts as one occurrence of the behavior. Because this is also time based, you will use the same "keep it simple" measurement strategies as duration.

Intensity

Tracking the intensity of a target behavior involves dividing the behavior into various degrees of intensity and using that to track any changes. The key to measuring intensity is the creation of a sound and reliable rating system. Consider the following example of an intensity scale for an individual who punches the wall:

> **Level 1**—pounds fist on wall
> **Level 2**—pounds fist on wall repeatedly
> **Level 3**—pounds fist on wall; makes hole
> **Level 4**—pounds fist on wall repeatedly;
> makes multiple holes (indicate number)

Examples of behaviors conducive to an intensity rating include episodes of aggression, tantrums, or property destruction, or behaviors such as screaming in which the volume changes.

When measuring intensity, you need to record the level of each occurrence. Note that when you measure intensity, you automatically get a count of frequency. Each intensity level that you record counts as one occurrence of the behavior. If you observe for different lengths of time each day, you will need to calculate a rate of occurrence of behaviors at each intensity level. To do this, divide the number of behaviors at each intensity level by the length of the observation period.

Keep It Simple Summary

In order to make this type of data collection practical, consider the following tricks.

- Wrap a piece of masking tape around your wrist and keep a marker in your pocket. Jot down the intensity rating on the tape each time the behavior occurs and then put the pen back in your pocket. At the end of the observation period, transfer data to data sheet.
- Either use a clipboard with the data sheet in Appendix D or keep the data sheet and pen close to where behavior occurs and jot down intensity level.

Using Samples of Behavior

All of the measurement approaches described above require the observer to pay attention throughout the entire observation period. Additionally, they are designed for behaviors that are somewhat discrete, in that a beginning and an end can be detected. Not all behaviors or situations are conducive to these approaches, however. Some behaviors may be nearly constant or may happen too rapidly for you to count each occurrence. Sometimes staff or family members have too many other demands to focus solely on one child and one behavior.

For these situations, a group of alternative approaches are available that rely on samples of behavior rather than constant observation. A sample is a little piece of something that represents the whole. For example, if you wanted to know the quality of the water in a reservoir, you wouldn't test every drop. Instead you would take out a little bit of the water and test that to give you a picture of what the whole reservoir is like. In calculating ratings of television shows, networks do not monitor every single person who watches television. Instead, they have boxes in a small group of people's homes that tell them what these viewers are watching and then they use this data to estimate what the entire population of television viewers prefers. Again, this is a sample of the behavior. We can use samples during functional behavior assessments too.

If a behavior is amenable to the measurement systems described above, but the team members do not have the freedom to observe and record the behavior accurately all day long, consider observing for a sample time interval. To do this, first you must identify whether you need to observe throughout the day or just during specified periods. If the behavior only occurs in certain settings (e.g., failure to respond to teacher instruction can only happen during periods of the day when teachers present instruction), then you already have natural limitations on when to observe. If the behavior is equally likely to happen at any time, it is best to spread out the periods of time that you observe. Let's say that you are a teacher, you are busy with other students, and cannot take detailed data on one student's behavior all day long, but the behavior does happen all day long. Choose three ten-minute periods of time throughout the day during which you will commit to keeping an eye on the student and measuring the behavior. You can use the same ten-minute periods of time each day or rotate through the day randomly to get a broader sample. During this period, you can record the behavior as you normally would have using the measure above that is best suited to the behavior along with the appropriate data sheet.

Some behaviors require different measurement strategies. These include behaviors:

- that do not have a clear beginning and end (e.g., near constant self-talk),
- that occur too quickly to count each one (e.g., hand flapping), or
- that happen too constantly throughout the day to count (e.g., constant humming).

Partial Interval Time Sample

One alternative available for behaviors like these is called a "partial interval time sample." When using this strategy, the observation period is broken into smaller intervals and the observer makes an indication at the end of each interval as to whether or not the behavior occurred at all during that interval. For example, if a student engages in near constant self-talk, we might ask the question, "During how many one-minute intervals per day does the student engage in self-talk?" We are not going to count how many times this behavior occurs during each interval. Instead, we will simply record whether or not the behavior happened at all during that time period.

The key to using this approach is to select a time period that is big enough that you are sure to capture the behavior and small enough to be sure that changes in the behavior can be seen. Identifying appropriate intervals takes practice and you may need to try out a couple of different intervals before committing to one for the full assessment. Or you can select a starting interval by spending one day measuring the time between occurrences of the behavior to identify the longest gap. Then set the observation interval a little smaller than that time period. So, if the child never goes more than ten minutes without self-talk, set your observation period at eight minutes.

To implement this strategy, buy a timer, set it for the appropriate interval, and then, when the timer goes off, use the Time Sample Data Sheet in Appendix E to record whether or not the problem behavior occurred during that interval.

Momentary Time Sample

A similar approach that is useful either for the highest frequency behaviors or for team members who cannot watch the individual with ASD through the whole observation period is called a "momentary time sample." This approach also involves identifying an appropriate interval but differs in that the observer only records what is going on at the end of that interval. If the behavior occurred fifteen times before the end of the interval, it does not matter. The only thing that is recorded is what is happening at the moment the interval ends.

To use this strategy, choose an appropriate interval as described in the section above. Then set a timer for the appropriate interval and look at the child when the timer goes off. Record whether or not the behavior is occurring at that moment. For this approach, it is best to use a vibrating timer so the child will not know when he is being observed.

For each of these measurement strategies, if each observation period lasts a different length of time, you will need to calculate a percent of intervals during which the behavior occurred. This will ensure that the numbers used to summarize performance are comparable.

Permanent Products

A final measure of behavior that is by far the simplest to use is referred to as permanent products. When relying on a permanent products measure, you assess naturally occurring, lasting records of a behavior. Some examples might include counting the number of worksheets a child completed, counting the number of holes a student punched in the wall, or counting the number of bite marks on someone's arm. The obvious advantage of this approach is that the data can be recorded long after the behavior is complete. This is especially advantageous for dangerous behaviors, as it frees up the caregiver to maintain safety and attend to the behavior at the time that it occurs rather than having to attend to measurement, without sacrificing measurement.

Of course, this approach will only work with behaviors that actually leave a permanent product. For example, you could not measure rocking with a permanent products measure. In contrast, breaking pencils in half would be conducive to this approach.

Refer to Appendix F for a Permanent Products data sheet.

Step 5: Establish a Baseline

The next step in the assessment process is to establish a baseline. A baseline is a quantitative measure of a behavior in its natural state. In other words, a baseline is a picture of what the behavior would look like if we never did anything specific to address it and we just kept doing whatever we'd been doing all along. For example, to establish a baseline of Jamaal's postures and faces, we would simply measure what he's doing without introducing any intervention. To establish a baseline of wisecracks for the student who made wisecracks in class, we would perhaps count the number of wisecracks.

A common misconception about establishing a baseline is that the behavior is measured while the adult ignores the child's behavior. This will not necessarily provide a baseline. If the adult was not previously ignoring the behavior, then we are not measuring the natural state of the behavior. Instead, we are measuring the behavior under the condition of being ignored. This may change the behavior. For example, imagine if Anthony's parents suddenly stopped giving Anthony his beads when he banged his head, thereby ignoring the behavior. Certainly, Anthony's behavior would change. Maybe his behavior would initially get worse because he was confused that his previously reinforced behavior was not getting reinforced. Maybe he would stop banging his head altogether. Maybe he would try something different to get the beads. We would get one picture of Anthony's behavior from this assessment, and as soon as baseline ended, and his parents stopped ignoring the behavior, the behavior would look totally different.

You may wonder why establishing a baseline is so critical. Baseline answers the following key questions:

1. What is the general level of the behavior? Measuring the behavior as part of a baseline gives the team a sense of how strong the behavior is. Many times, measuring baseline allows a team to see that a behavior is not as intrusive as they once thought. Sometimes a very disturbing behavior can happen just once or twice and because the nature of the behavior is upsetting, it seems that an intervention is urgently necessary. Nevertheless, the baseline data reveals that the behavior is really very rare and not a priority at all. Establishing a baseline can prevent teams from devoting a great deal of time and energy to a low-level behavior.

Conversely, baseline data may be helpful in convincing a skeptical team member that an intervention is, in fact, necessary when the data show the consistency or high level of the behavior. The sample graph below illustrates a low-level behavior. If this graph were measuring a highly intrusive behavior, such as aggression, even this low level might be too high and call for intervention. However, if the behavior being measured has less significant effects, such as humming or nail-biting, this behavior may not warrant any intervention, as it is very infrequent.

2. Is the behavior getting stronger, weaker, or staying the same? Measuring a baseline allows us to see the direction that a behavior is taking. If a behavior is getting worse or staying at a high level, then further assessment, and, ultimately, an intervention is warranted. However, sometimes baseline data reveals that a behavior problem is resolving on its own. Whatever environmental variables are in place are exactly what is needed for the behavior to go away. In this case, changing the environment by introducing an intervention would present a risk that the behavior would instead get stronger. Because the purpose of an assessment is to inform intervention, there is no need for intervention in that scenario.

Occasionally, a behavior might be weakening, but at too slow a pace. In this case, team members may decide that an intervention is worthwhile, all the while acknowledging the risk of derailing the ongoing improvements. To determine the direction of the behavior, baseline must last long enough to demonstrate patterns of the behavior. One common strategy is to gather 3 to 5 "data points"; that is, to measure the behavior on 3 to 5 separate occasions. However, this guideline only applies when a pattern is evident within that time period. You may need to extend baseline if a pattern is not evident by that point. The graph below illustrates a response that is increasing. If this graph represented a maladaptive behavior, then an intervention would certainly be warranted.

Sample Baseline Data: Increasing Trend

3. Is the behavior consistent or variable? Measuring a baseline allows team members to determine whether or not a behavior is stable. If the behavior is at a pretty consistent level or is following a pretty consistent growth curve, then the team can be assured that the variables that affect the behavior are consistent across settings. If the behavior is variable, meaning that it is sometimes very strong and sometimes very weak, then that gives us a clue that something specific to certain settings or contexts is affecting the behavior. It can be beneficial to give variable behaviors some time to stabilize before intervening, as it might turn out that when a trend is finally apparent, the behavior is decreasing.

The graph below illustrates a behavior with a highly variable pattern. Note that in order to figure out what is going on, labeling the data points is critical. This enables even the most variable data to tell a coherent story.

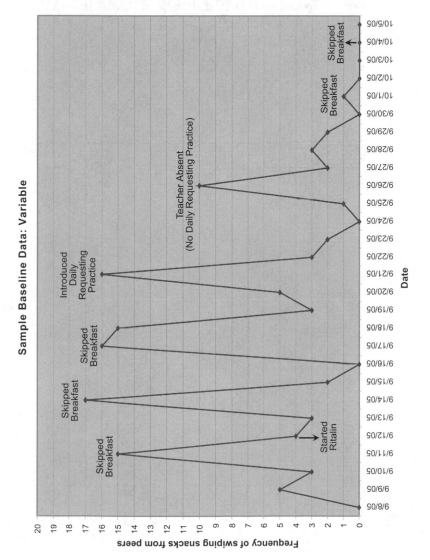

Keep It Simple Summary

To establish a baseline, measure a behavior while doing whatever you've been doing all along. If it turns out to be a low intensity, low-level behavior, or if the behavior turns out to be decreasing, continue measuring the behavior until it is gone. No other forms of intervention are necessary. If the behavior is very variable, try to identify variables that are in place when the behavior is stronger or weaker. Possible variables include: the people who are interacting with the individual, the time of day, changes in medication, etc.

5 | Finding Out Who Knows What

You have assembled a team of people knowledgeable about the problem behavior you wish to target. At this point in the process, it is time to find out what they know. While you may feel that chatting informally with someone is sufficient, you risk omitting important questions if you don't do a structured interview. Furthermore, you may not allow the interviewee enough time to focus on the behavior problem if you do not create a scenario in which he or she can concentrate on the behavior.

Step 6: Interview Team Members

When you interview someone as part of a functional behavior assessment, your goal is to identify patterns in the behavior that will help you identify the behavior's function or functions. Thinking back to how behaviors are learned will help you figure out what you need to ask your interviewees. Specifically, you will want to ask questions that help you determine the following types of information:

- The immediate antecedent and consequences of the behavior.
- What the individual has access to (or escapes from) after performing the behavior that she didn't have access to (or the ability to escape from) before.
- Any establishing operations that may be in effect. (Does the behavior occur after a long period of deprivation

from something preferred? Or does it occur after a long period of interaction with something non-preferred?)

- If different reporters describe different environmental conditions when the behavior occurs, or if the same behavior patterns are recurring in different settings.
- How well the individual communicates and the consequences of appropriate communication.

To help get at these questions, a blank, reproducible interview questionnaire is included on the next page. Guidelines for interpreting responses to the questions are also provided.

When interviewing team members, there are a few strategies to keep in mind. First of all, you are looking for facts rather than opinions. The goal of the assessment is to develop and test hypotheses based on facts. This will lead to a more accurate and efficient assessment. Separate opinion from fact whenever possible. For example, if someone says, "I'm sure he's doing this to get attention," that is clearly an opinion. Follow up with a fact-finding question such as, "Tell me some of your observations that have led you to feel this way" or "How can you tell?" If your reporter responds by saying something like, "He checks to see if I'm looking whenever he does it," that sounds more like a fact.

Because people's opinions tend to skew their observations and consequently their reporting, it is important to interview multiple reporters. If few reporters are available, feel free to answer the questions in the interview yourself. Try to do this before interviewing anyone else so that your answers are not influenced by others. Also, to protect your interviewees from being swayed by one another, try to interview them individually.

The benefit of using the questions below as an interview rather than as a written questionnaire is that you can follow up on certain answers or clarify certain responses. However, there are times when it will not be feasible to interview each team member who might have valuable information. In those cases, feel free to give them the list of questions to respond to as a questionnaire. Administered as an interview, the following questions will require approximately thirty minutes to complete, depending on the amount of information available.

Functional Behavior Assessment Interview Form

Behavior:_____

Definition of Behavior:

_____

_____

_____

Date: _____

Interviewer (individual asking the questions):_____

Reporter (individual answering the questions): _____

Instructions to Interviewer:
1. Begin by introducing self and role, if necessary.
2. Label target behavior and read definition to interviewee. Before beginning interview, confirm that interviewee has seen the behavior. If yes, proceed with interview. If no, but the person does have other information about the individual who is exhibiting the problem behavior, please ask only those questions relevant to "background information" and "communication skills."
3. Explain to the interviewee that he or she may not have the information to answer each question (e.g., a teacher may not have information about sleep patterns). Ask each question anyway in case they have information that you might not expect.
4. Be sure to solicit examples whenever possible with the goal of distinguishing fact from opinion.

Background Information
1. What is your role in relation to [   ] *(individual's name)*?

_____

2. How long have you known [   ]? _____
3. Does [   ] have a consistent schedule (each day or on some days)? _____
4. If yes, please describe. _____

_____

(Continued on next page.)

5. Does [   ] have a sense of this schedule? Does he or she know what comes next? _____

6. What are [   ]'s favorite things (objects, people, and activities) in this setting? _____

   a. In what situations are these things earned?

   _____

   b. In what situations does [   ] have free access to these things?

   _____

   c. In what situations does [   ] have little or no access to these things?

   _____

   d. For those who have seen the behavior problem: Does the behavior problem vary in each of the above situations?

   _____

7. What are [   ]'s least favorite things (objects, people, and activities)? _____

   a. In what situations does [   ] have inescapable exposure to these things? _____

   _____

   b. In what situations does [   ] have escapable exposure to these things? _____

   _____

   c. In what situations does [   ] have no contact with these things at all? _____

   _____

   d. For those who have seen the behavior problem: Does the behavior problem vary in each of the above situations?

   _____

8. Does [   ] have peers/siblings with whom he or she enjoys interacting? _____

9. Are there adults with whom [   ] enjoys interacting?

   _____

10. How much access to social interaction does [   ] have throughout the day? _____

11. Is [   ] well liked by peers/siblings? _____

12. Is [   ] well liked by adults? _____

(Continued on next page.)

13. How does [   ] respond to difficult tasks?

_____

14. How does [   ] respond to interrupting desired activities?

_____

15. How does [   ] respond to withdrawal of attention?

_____

16. How does [   ] respond to sharing attention with someone else? _____

_____

Communication Skills

1. How does [   ] make his or her wants and needs known?

_____

2. What is the easiest means of communication for [   ]?

_____

3. How does [   ] obtain your attention?

_____

   • What percent of time (approx.) do you provide attention in response to this bid? _____

4. How does [   ] let you know when he/she wants to socialize with you? _____

   • What percent of time (approx.) does this bid result in socialization? _____

5. How does [   ] let you know when he/she wants an object or activity? _____

   • What percent of time (approx.) do you provide the object or activity in response to this bid? _____

6. How does [   ] request a break from tasks or a different task? _____

   • What percent of time (approx.) do you provide a break or new task in response to this bid? _____

History of Behavior

1. When did you first notice the target behavior? _____

_____

(Continued on next page.)

2. Were there any changes that you know of that coincided with the onset of the behavior? _____

_____

    a. Were any new demands placed on [   ]?

    _____

    b. Were any demands on [   ] increased?

    _____

    c. Were demands removed or reduced?

    _____

    d. Did the ratio of children to caregivers change at that time?

    _____

    e. Did any children enter or leave the environment at that time?

    _____

    f. Did any adults enter or leave the environment at that time?

    _____

    g. Was the level of attention altered in any way at that time?

    _____

    h. Did [   ]'s schedule or activities change at that time? _____

    i. Did the available materials change at that time? _____

    j. Was there any illness at that time? _____

    k. Was there any medication change at that time? _____

    l. Was there any change in sleep patterns at that time?

    _____

    m. Was there any change in eating patterns at that time?

    _____

    n. Was there any change in [   ]'s physical environment at that time? _____

Present Picture of the Behavior

1. How often do you see the behavior? _____

2. Is it likely to occur with any other behaviors? _____

3. Are there certain situations in which the behavior always occurs?

_____

(Continued on next page.)

4. Are there certain situations in which the behavior never occurs?

_____

5. Can you elicit the behavior? If yes, how? _____

6. Can you prevent the behavior? If yes, how? _____

7. Is the behavior more intense in some circumstances? If yes, when?

_____

8. Is the behavior milder in some circumstances? If yes, when?

_____

9. Are there certain days of the week the behavior is more or less likely to occur? _____

   • If yes, what is different about [   ]'s schedule on those days? _____

10. Are there certain times of day that the behavior is more or less likely to occur? _____

   • If yes, what is going on in [   ]'s schedule at that time? _____

11. Are there certain settings in which the behavior is more or less likely to occur? _____

12. Are there certain people with whom the behavior is more or less likely to occur? _____

13. Are there certain activities during which the behavior is more or less likely to occur? _____

14. Are there certain materials that are usually present when the behavior occurs? _____

15. Are there certain materials that are usually not present when the behavior occurs? _____

16. Have you noticed any common triggers for the behavior?

_____

17. How do you usually respond to the behavior?

_____

18. How do others usually respond to the behavior?

_____

19. Do you think the behavior would happen if [   ] were left alone? _____

20. Have you ever walked in on [   ] performing the behavior when he or she was alone? _____

(Continued on next page.)

Physiological Considerations

1. What medications is [   ] taking right now?

   _____

2. When did [   ] start taking this medication?

   _____

3. What are some common side effects? _____

   _____

4. Why is he or she taking this medication? _____

   _____

5. Does [   ] have any illnesses or conditions?

   _____

   • If yes, do you notice any relationship between [   ]'s
   behavior and the severity of these conditions? _____

6. Describe [   ]'s sleep patterns. _____

   _____

   • Do you notice any relationship between [   ]'s
   sleep and behavior? _____

7. Describe [   ]'s eating patterns. _____

   _____

   • Do you notice any relationship between [   ]'s
   eating and behavior? _____

Functional Behavior Assessment Interview Form
INTERPRETATION GUIDE

Background Information

1. What is your role in relation to [   ] *(individual's name)*?
   Use response to determine areas of interviewee's expertise.

2. How long have you known [   ]?
   Use response to estimate level of interviewee's expertise.

3. Does [   ] have a consistent schedule (each day or on some days)?

4. If yes, please describe.
   Use schedule as a reference for baseline data. Compare levels of behavior when the individual has different activities scheduled. Also, compare description of schedule among different respondents. If descriptions conflict, schedule probably varies based on who is with the individual.

5. Does [   ] have a sense of this schedule? Does he or she know what comes next?
   If target behavior consistently occurs prior to a certain activity, possibly delaying it, the individual may be avoiding this activity if he/she is able to predict schedule.

6. What are [   ]'s favorite things *(objects, people, and activities)* in this setting?
   Does interviewee know what learner's favorite things are? If no, learner may not have enough access to preferences. Learner also may not be able to communicate preferences. Enriching learner's environment by adding preferred objects and activities, as well as other types of stimulation, may decrease target behavior.

   a. In what situations are these things earned?

   b. In what situations does [   ] have free access to these things?

   c. In what situations does [   ] have little or no access to these things?

   d. For those who have seen the behavior problem: Does the behavior problem vary in each of the above situations?

   These questions are all designed to give clues about the level of enrichment and the relationship between access to

(Continued on next page.)

preferred items and behavior problems. Lower levels of enrichment might be associated with automatic reinforcement behaviors, as [   ] has nothing else to do, and thereby "entertains" him- or herself with the target behavior. Relatively high behavior problems in situations with restricted access to preferred items or activities suggest that automatic reinforcement might be the function of the behavior.

7. What are [   ]'s least favorite things (objects, people, and activities)?

    a. In what situations does [   ] have inescapable exposure to these things?

    b. In what situations does [   ] have escapable exposure to these things?

    c. In what situations does [   ] have no contact with these things at all?

    d. For those who have seen the behavior problem: Does the behavior problem vary in each of the above situations?

    These questions are all designed to give clues about possible escape behaviors. Also, too much exposure to aversive situations signals the need for an enriched environment. For more on intervention strategies, see Chapter 8.

8. Does [   ] have peers/siblings with whom he or she enjoys interacting?

9. Are there adults with whom [   ] enjoys interacting?

10. How much access to social interaction does [   ] have throughout the day?
These questions are geared to assessing the level of attention that the individual has each day, as well as whether or not attention is a motivator for this child.

11. Is [   ] well liked by peers/siblings?

12. Is [   ] well liked by adults?
When learners are not well liked, they typically receive a lower quality or quantity of attention. This might be associated with problem behaviors maintained by attention (i.e., the individual may be engaging in the problem behavior so that others will pay attention to him or her).

13. How does [   ] respond to difficult tasks?
To assess possible escape-maintained behaviors.

(Continued on next page.)

14. How does [   ] respond to interrupting desired activities?
    To assess behaviors maintained by access to objects or activities.

15. How does [   ] respond to withdrawal of attention?
    To assess behaviors maintained by attention.

16. How does [   ] respond to sharing attention with someone else?
    To assess behaviors maintained by attention.

Communication Skills

1. How does [   ] make his or her wants and needs known?

2. What is the easiest means of communication for [   ]?

3. How does [   ] obtain your attention?

    • What percent of time (approx.) do you provide attention in response to this bid?

4. How does [   ] let you know when he/she wants to socialize with you?

    • What percent of time (approx.) does this bid result in socialization?

5. How does [   ] let you know when he/she wants an object or activity?

    • What percent of time (approx.) do you provide the object or activity in response to this bid?

6. How does [   ] request a break from tasks or a different task?

    • What percent of time (approx.) do you provide a break or new task in response to this bid?

All of the above questions are geared toward assessing the efficiency of using appropriate versus inappropriate behaviors to obtain what is wanted. If a deficit in communication skills is identified, an intervention might focus on building skills in this arena rather than addressing the target behavior directly.

History of Behavior

1. When did you first notice the target behavior?
   This question helps assess how long the behavior has been a problem in this particular setting. By interviewing multiple

(Continued on next page.)

informants, it is possible to determine where the behavior first appeared. This may offer a clue as to the function. If a behavior problem has been around so long that the staff members cannot recall when the behavior began, that just suggests that it might take a little longer for the intervention to work, as the behavior has such a long learning history to "unlearn." Just skip the following section and move on.

2. Were there any changes that you know of that coincided with the onset of the behavior?

    a. Were any new demands placed on [   ]?

    b. Were any demands on [   ] increased?
       To assess a possible escape function of the behavior.

    c. Were demands removed or reduced?
       Unstructured time is often very demanding for people with autism. This question therefore assesses behaviors related to escape from the demand of needing to fill one's own time or sitting quietly, etc. Also, a sudden increase in downtime might be associated with an increase in automatic reinforcement behaviors.

    d. Did the ratio of children to caregivers change at that time?

    e. Did any children enter or leave the environment at that time?

    f. Did any adults enter or leave the environment at that time?

    g. Was the level of attention altered in any way at that time?
       These questions are geared toward assessing attention-related variables. A behavior problem may also involve escape from the attention of a non-preferred person.

    h. Did [   ]'s schedule or activities change at that time?

    i. Did the available materials change at that time?
       These questions are geared toward assessing behaviors related to objects and activities.

    j. Was there any illness at that time?

    k. Was there any medication change at that time?

    l. Was there any change in sleep patterns at that time?

    m. Was there any change in eating patterns at that time?
       These questions are geared toward assessing any physiological factors affecting the behavior. These can either alter someone's threshold for behavior "shortening

(Continued on next page.)

their fuse," so to speak, or may be associated with automatic reinforcement behaviors. This information will also help clarify whether or not a certain behavior problem may be a side effect of a medication.

n. Was there any change in [   ]'s physical environment at that time?
This question is geared toward assessing whether the individual may be responding to some sort of stimulation from the physical environment, either escaping an unwanted sensation, or reacting to a higher level of distraction, etc.

Present Picture of the Behavior

1. How often do you see the behavior?
The answer to this, along with baseline data, allows comparison across settings.

2. Is it likely to occur with any other behaviors?
The answer to this allows hypothesis for other behaviors that might serve the same function. For example, if head-hitting and hand-biting usually occur together, they are likely to serve the same function

3. Are there certain situations in which the behavior always occurs?

4. Are there certain situations in which the behavior never occurs?
Identify characteristics of each setting as a clue to the function of the behavior. For example, if it always happens during work and never during breaks, it is probably escape related.

5. Can you elicit the behavior? If yes, how?
This answer will specify at least one of the immediate antecedents.

6. Can you prevent the behavior? If yes, how?
Identifying variables that prevent a behavior gives clues to motivation. For example, if behavior can be prevented by seating the child alone, behavior may occur to escape attention.

7. Is the behavior more intense in some circumstances? If yes, when?

8. Is the behavior milder in some circumstances? If yes, when?

9. Are there certain days of the week the behavior is more or less likely to occur?

   • If yes, what is different about [   ]'s schedule on those days?

10. Are there certain times of day that the behavior is more or less likely to occur?

(Continued on next page.)

• If yes, what is going on in [   ]'s schedule at
that time?

11. Are there certain settings in which the behavior is more or less
likely to occur?

12. Are there certain people with whom the behavior is more or less
likely to occur?

13. Are there certain activities during which the behavior is more or
less likely to occur?

14. Are there certain materials that are usually present when the
behavior occurs?

15. Are there certain materials that are usually not present when the
behavior occurs?
*The task, when considering answers to all of the above, is to identify
the variables that do and do not lead to the behavior. Think about
the people who are around when the behavior occurs. What do
they do differently than the people with whom the behavior does not
occur? Do they offer a richer quality of attention when the child is
on-task? Do they offer more consistent contingencies (i.e., reinforce-
ent? punishment?) for inappropriate behavior? Alternatively, they
may not place as many demands on the child. They may give her
free access to preferred items or activities. Observations of each of
these contrasts would lead you toward a different intervention.
Sometimes differences in the individual's behavior with different
people are not due to these individuals' behaviors. Perhaps an
instructor associated with greater behavior problems wears a
certain perfume that the student attempts to escape from. Maybe
one instructor's voice is louder than another's and leads to escape
behaviors. In any case, you can see how identifying the specific
variable associated with the behavior problem will guide intervention.
Similarly, identifying specific environmental variables
associated with the problem behavior will guide intervention.
Consider lighting, smells, textures, tastes, temperature, crowded-
ness, volume, etc. in each environment where the behavior does and
does not occur. If you can isolate a variable that is common to
settings where the behavior occurs and is absent from settings
where the behavior does not occur, then you are on the path to
effective intervention.*

16. Have you noticed any common triggers for the behavior?
Identifies immediate antecedents.

17. How do you usually respond to the behavior?
Identifies consequences.

(Continued on next page.)

18. How do others usually respond to the behavior?
    Identifies consequences.

19. Do you think the behavior would happen if [   ] were left alone?

20. Have you ever walked in on [   ] performing the behavior when he or she was alone?
    If the behavior occurs when the learner is left alone, this suggests automatically reinforced behavior—unless it occurs because no one is present to stop it (e.g., stealing cookies).

Physiological Considerations

1. What medications is [   ] taking right now?

2. When did [   ] start taking this medication?

3. What are some common side effects?

4. Why is he or she taking this medication?

5. Does [   ] have any illnesses or conditions?

    • If yes, do you notice any relationship between [   ]'s behavior and the severity of these conditions?

6. Describe [   ]'s sleep patterns.

    • Do you notice any relationship between [   ]'s sleep and behavior?

7. Describe [   ]'s eating patterns.

    • Do you notice any relationship between [   ]'s eating and behavior?

These questions are geared toward assessing any physiological factors affecting the behavior. These can either alter someone's threshold for behavior—"shortening their fuse," so to speak, or may be associated with automatic reinforcement behaviors. This information will also help clarify whether or not a certain behavior problem may be a side effect of a medication.

SAMPLE
Functional Behavior Assessment Interview
for Students

Behavior: _____

Definition of Behavior: _____

_____

_____

_____

Date: _____

Interviewer (individual asking the questions):_____

Reporter (individual answering the questions): _____

[Interviewer: Adjust wording of questions according to child's age.]

1. When are you most likely to (problem behavior)? _____

_____

   a. Are there times that you are sure you would? _____

   b. Are there times that you are sure you wouldn't? _____

2. When is it the hardest to resist doing (problem behavior)?

_____

3. What could we do to help you not (problem behavior)?

_____

4. How do you let people know when something is too hard for you?

_____

   • How do they respond? _____

5. How do you let people know when something is too boring for you?

_____

   • How do they respond? _____

(Continued on next page.)

6. How do you let people know when you need a break?

   _____

   • How do they respond? _____

7. How do you let people know when you need help?

   _____

   • How do they respond? _____

8. How do you let people know when you need some attention?

   _____

   • How do they respond? _____

9. How do you let people know when you need some space?

   _____

   • How do they respond? _____

10. How do you let people know when you'd like to do a certain activity?

    _____

    • How do they respond? _____

11. How does it feel to you when you do (problem behavior)?

    _____

12. In general, would you describe your work as too hard, too easy, or just right?

    _____

13. In general, do you feel that people notice when you do a good job?

    _____

14. What are your favorite things to do? When do you get to do these?

    _____

15. What are your least favorite things to do? When do you have to do these?

    _____

16. Is there anything we could do to change your least favorite activities?

    _____

6 | Observation Time

Up until this point, you have been gathering the tools that you'll need to investigate the seemingly senseless behavior of your child or student. Finally, you are ready to use these tools to investigate the behavior's function. Specifically, you will use systematic observation to try to identify EO's, immediate antecedents, and consequences that may be at play. This chapter will describe several approaches to observation commonly used in functional behavior assessments.

Step 7: Observe the Behavior

Listed below are several observational tools that can help unearth clues. You will not need to use all of these approaches in a single investigation. However, having information about each of them will allow you to choose one or more strategies to employ.

Unstructured Observation

This approach is exactly what it sounds like: You will take some time to pull yourself out of the situation and watch the behavior, along with its context. Stepping back in this way is critical because it is nearly impossible to get a clear picture of the influencing variables while interacting with your child.

While observing, ask yourself all of the questions included in the interview. For example, try to notice what happened just before the behavior and what happened just after the behavior. Try to identify what your child might have wanted, along with what he got. Make note of who is always around when the behavior occurs, and with whom the behavior is consistently absent. What do these individuals do differently with your child? Also notice during which activity the behavior occurs and which materials are being used at the time, as well as whether or not the context seems to affect the behavior.

Sometimes it is not possible to watch without altering your child's behavior (perhaps because he only does the behavior with you), or you may simply not have enough people around at the time that the behavior usually occurs to pull yourself away. If you are in this situation, consider setting up a video camera and trying to catch the behavior on tape. You can watch the tape later and get the same information from the video.

It is surprising how informative a simple peek at what is happening can be. Many times, patterns will jump out at you that will make the function of the behavior clear. For example, a behavior may occur consistently whenever a sibling enters the room. Or maybe the behavior occurs whenever it's time to put away a preferred activity. Sometimes your child will give you a clue while he is in the midst of the behavior, such as looking at someone's face for a certain response. Sometimes you might notice a consistent consequence. The more occurrences of the behavior you see, the more information you'll have. Try to see the behavior about ten times as a bare minimum, although guidelines for infrequent yet severe behaviors are presented later in the "Special Considerations" section in Chapter 9 of this book.

Unstructured observation is a great way to develop hypotheses about the function of a behavior. You should spend some time doing unstructured observation as a first step in every functional behavior assessment. However, because there is no data collection to confirm or refute any hypotheses that develop, you must always use another observational strategy in conjunction with this one before completing your assessment.

Structured Observation

In addition to using unstructured observation to gain information about the function of a behavior, it is often extremely useful to observe behavior very systematically. The main observation tools that are used for structured observations are: A-B-C Data and Descriptive Analysis.

A-B-C Data

"A-B-C" data stands for "Antecedent-Behavior-Consequence." As you might guess, the purpose of identifying A-B-C patterns is to develop hypotheses about what exactly has been learned about the problem behavior. We can identify the behavior's function by identifying consequences that reverse antecedents (e.g., A = teacher walks away from student, B = problem behavior, C = teacher returns to student to redirect). Similarly, by identifying consistent pairings between antecedents and consequences, we might identify events that act as S^D's for the behavior. For example, imagine a child who always cries for candy when his grandmother comes over and then is given some candy. For this child, Grandma may be an S^D signaling the availability of candy. Consider the following examples on the chart on the next page and then try to complete the blank spaces in the chart on your own.

Notice in the examples that each antecedent is a discrete event. The immediate antecedent is whatever changed in the environment just as the behavior occurred. These events may either trigger EO's or serve as S^D's for the problem behavior.

Individuals new to A-B-C data collection commonly make the mistake of describing a setting or ongoing activity rather than identifying an antecedent. For example, for number 5, if the antecedent had been listed as "play with mom," the function of the behavior would have been less clear. For number 1, if the antecedent had been listed as "classroom," again the function of the behavior would have been less clear. It is sometimes challenging to identify relevant discrete changes in the environment that precede a behavior, but doing so will lead to much clearer assessment information. With

Example Number	Antecedent	Behavior	Consequence	Possible Function(s)
1	"Time for Work"	Mia pounds her fist on her desk	Time out in hallway	Escape task
2	Peer approach and greeting	Mia pounds her fist on her desk	Peer walks away	Escape peer interaction
3	Alone, no demands, no specific activity	Mia pounds her fist on her desk	Alone, no demands, no specific activity	Automatic reinforcement
4	Alone, no demands, no specific activity	Mia pounds her fist on her desk	Sent for therapeutic brushing	Automatic reinforcement; access to brushing
5	Mom interrupts play with Mia to answer ringing phone	Mia pounds her fist on her desk	Mom hangs up to attend to problem behavior	Obtain attention
6	Peer greets another peer	Mia pounds her fist on her desk	Peers laugh and smile at Mia	
7	Instructor says, "Do this" and presents model for imitation	Mia pounds her fist on her desk	Instructor restrains Mia	
8	Dad shuts light, says, "good night"	Mia pounds her fist on her desk	Mia alone in room in dark	

Answers:
6. Obtain peer attention
7. Escape task; obtain physical attention
8. Automatic reinforcement

practice, identifying these discrete antecedents becomes easier. To help the observer distinguish between settings, ongoing activities, and immediate antecedents, each of these categories are included on the A-B-C Data Sheet in Appendix G.

Another error that individuals new to A-B-C data often make involves drawing conclusions from too few A-B-C sequences. To suggest that a behavior has a certain function, A-B-C data needs to show a pattern repeatedly. To help identify predominant patterns in your A-B-C data, you will be asked to total the number of times that each possible function arises at the bottom of your data sheet. If one possible function emerges much more often than others, you have some evidence to suggest that it might be influencing the behavior.

If possible, try to have more than one person collect A-B-C data as well as evaluate the data as to possible functions. Unfortunately, recent research findings suggest that different raters of A-B-C data do not always agree with one another (Kwak, Ervin, Anderson, & Austin, 2004). This tells us that the same set of data may be interpreted differently by different raters. If you can have another person review your data and your ratings agree, this makes your findings particularly compelling. Nevertheless, it will still be best to pursue confirmation of these findings through another observation method.

Descriptive Analysis

A descriptive analysis involves comparing the strength of the behavior under different naturally occurring conditions. Using this method requires the observer to quickly recognize the controlling factors in place. The observer must be able to identify the answers to each of the following questions on a moment-to-moment basis:

1. Is there a demand on the learner?
2. Is he receiving attention?
3. Is his access to a desired item or activity restricted?

It may be helpful to use your knowledge of the child's daily routine to try to plan times to observe under four conditions:

1. high demands,
2. low attention,
3. restricted access to things he likes, and
4. free access to preferred items and attention.

If this is not possible, don't worry. You can also watch any time and sort out which of the above conditions were in place.

If the situations that you'd like to observe (i.e., low attention, high demands, and restricted access) do not occur naturally, you may have to ask the adult who will be interacting with the child to set these situations up. However, keep in mind that this does not guarantee that those conditions will be in place. For example, you may ask a teacher to place demands on a student, but the demands might get derailed by off-task behavior. An adult may provide constant eye contact to a student he is supposed to be ignoring.

These observations provide extremely valuable information for your assessment regarding both the impact of the child's behavior on his environment and the way that others in that environment respond to him. Observe and decide what conditions are in place.

The observer then uses his or her measurement tools to record the strength of the behavior under each condition.(Refer back to Chapter 4 for information on measuring behaviors.) By calculating the average strength of the behavior under each condition, the observer gathers evidence as to what the function(s) of the behavior might be. For example, if a behavior is much more likely to occur when someone places a particular type of demand on the individual, then the behavior is likely to serve as an escape from that particular type of demand. If the behavior occurs more frequently when the individual is not receiving attention, then the behavior may function to obtain attention. If the behavior occurs whenever access to a desired item is restricted, then the behavior may operate to get the item back.

Sometimes, behaviors occur fairly equally across all conditions. In this case, either the behavior actually serves each function, or the behavior is automatically reinforcing. To help flesh this out, try observing your child when he is alone. If the behavior often occurs when he is alone, there is a good chance that the behavior serves an automatic reinforcement function. Nothing in the external environment is changing, but the behavior occurs anyway. Immediate antecedents and reinforcers for the behavior are taking place internally. Alternatively, if the behavior does not occur when your child is alone, consider his communication skills and whether or not appropriate requests are reinforced.

If your child's communication skills need to be developed, and/or appropriate requests are unlikely to be reinforced, then it is likely that the seemingly senseless behavior actually serves multiple functions.

In order to simplify the observation and interpretation process, a Descriptive Analysis Data Sheet is included in Appendix H.

7 | Test Your Hypothesis

After using one or more of the observational methods described in the previous chapter, you will have one or more hypotheses about the function of your child's behavior. Now is the time to test your hypotheses to see whether you are correct. To do so, you can use one of two methods in which you try to deliberately manipulate conditions so that your child engages in the problem behavior.

Step 8: Experiment with the Behavior

Below are systematic scientific procedures designed to help you isolate variables that may be contributing to behavior problems. With these strategies, you will not just record and categorize naturally occurring behavior, you will actually attempt to elicit the problem behavior, and, in some cases, reinforce it.

For less complex behaviors, it is usually sufficient to try to use antecedent manipulations first (see below). This assessment approach is easier to implement correctly, can be completed quickly, and will provide sufficient information to address most behavior problems. For more complex behaviors, a functional analysis may be warranted. This is the "gold standard" of assessment tools and can help shed light on even the most puzzling behavior problems. However, as this is more complicated and requires eliciting and reinforcing more of the challenging behavior, you may need the help of a professional to implement this approach, at least the first couple of times that you use it.

Importantly, before you use any of the techniques described that involve eliciting the behavior (i.e., setting up scenarios in which the behavior is likely to occur), consider the safety of everyone involved. Do not trigger dangerous behaviors without taking any necessary precautions first. For example, you may need something as intensive as asking a professional trained in crisis management to be present, or you may need something simple, like seating the caregiver near the door so that a quick exit is possible if behaviors escalate.

Antecedent Manipulation

Like descriptive analysis, antecedent manipulation involves comparing the strength of the behavior under different environmental conditions. However, in contrast to descriptive analysis, antecedent manipulation involves contriving situations to observe rather than waiting for events to take place naturally. Therefore, to use antecedent manipulation, the observer must actively set up different conditions to evaluate.

You can use antecedent manipulations to test any hypotheses that you may have developed during unstructured observation or descriptive analysis. These may or may not be more specific than one of the four classic functions:

1. Attention,
2. Objects and activities,
3. Escape/avoid, and
4. Automatic reinforcement.

For example, you might test "divided attention" rather than "low attention," or you might test "social demands" rather than "academic demands."

Alternatively, if you are really unsure of what the function of the behavior might be, or you suspect it might serve multiple functions, you can use antecedent manipulations to examine all four typical functions.

Some examples of more specific functions (not an exhaustive list):

1. Preventing divided attention,
2. Escape from social demands,
3. Escape from certain difficulty of instruction,
4. Escape from people who provide only low levels of unenthused attention,
5. Escape from loud, intrusive attention,
6. Escape from a certain odor,
7. Escape from crowds,
8. Access a certain individual's attention,
9. Access physical attention,
10. Escape tasks with non-preferred materials.

Whatever conditions you choose to test, you will also want to include a "control" condition. A "control" condition is designed to provide a contrast to the other conditions. It is meant to be a condition where you are unlikely to see the problem behavior. When implementing a control condition, rich levels of attention should be available to the child. Try to make it the type of attention that the child seems to prefer. When you are not sure whether or not the child wants your attention, offer a cue about every thirty seconds that your attention is available, such as praise or a comment based on what she is doing. Additionally, free access to lots of preferred objects and activities should be provided, and you should place no demands on the child at this time. With the exception of behavior problems that serve an automatic reinforcement function, you are unlikely to see behavior problems during a control condition. Even automatically reinforcing behaviors are less likely to occur during a control condition because competing reinforcers are available.

Preparing to Use Antecedent Manipulation

The following steps will guide you through preparing to use the antecedent manipulation strategy to test hypotheses about behavior.

1) Set Up Your Team

The antecedent manipulation strategy is designed to be implemented with one person interacting with the child and another person observing and recording data. It is possible, though less desirable, for one person to fill both roles. If you really can't get the help, or if you feel that having someone observe and record will alter the child's behavior, then it is possible to surreptitiously record the data while you interact with the child.

The downside of doing this solo is that you miss out on the opportunity to observe the whole interaction, and may have difficulty recording, observing, and interacting all at the same time. You may need to rely heavily on some of the tips for simplifying data collection described in Chapter 4, such as moving a penny from your left to your right pocket each time you observe the behavior. If you are implementing a low attention condition, be careful not to make it obvious that you are watching the child. As an alternative, consider videotaping a session with the camera on a tripod and scoring it later.

Sometimes, you may really need more than two people to test your ideas. For example, if you believe the behavior occurs due to divided attention or crowds, more participants will be required.

2) Choose How Long Each Test Condition Should Last

Each condition, including the control condition, must be introduced for the same amount of time. Typically, about ten minutes in each condition is enough to gather helpful information about the behavior. You may be able to gather information about a high frequency behavior with a shorter latency in only five minutes. Alternatively, a behavior that requires a longer period of deprivation to elicit or has a lower frequency might require fifteen- or twenty-minute sessions.

In extreme cases of severe, but low frequency behaviors, I have used conditions that last most of a school day. For example, I used a full-school-day assessment condition for a student who banged his head against hard surfaces so forcefully that he needed to wear a helmet to prevent serious injury. At times, the student removed the helmet to bang his head. Some staff members who worked with the student felt that he used this behavior to obtain sensory input (automatic reinforcement). Others felt that the behavior was related to the type of tasks that he was asked to do (escape from tasks). A-B-C data, interview, and observation were inconclusive. Because the behavior was infrequent, it was difficult to gather enough empirical information about antecedents and consequences to confirm either hypothesis.

In order to sort out and effectively treat this student's severe and dangerous behavior, we set up an entire school day for him in the control condition; an entire school day practicing repetitive and non-functional tasks (sorting random items, dumping them out, and sorting them again); and an entire school day practicing naturalistic and functional tasks (sorting dishes and putting them away). Then we repeated each day. The head-banging behavior only occurred in the condition involving repetitive and non-functional tasks. Consequently, we could clearly identify the function as escaping these tasks, and our direction for intervention was clear. If we had only had ten minutes in each of these conditions, a low frequency behavior such as this one may not have occurred, and we would not have been able to pinpoint the function and identify an effective treatment.

3) Choose the Conditions You Would Like to Test

Depending on what your hypotheses are regarding the function of the behavior, you will need to establish different conditions. The adult who will be interacting with the individual with ASD during the assessment must be taught how to set up the conditions and be provided with guidelines directing him how to behave in each condition. These guidelines for how to use antecedent manipulation to test each of the four classic hypotheses are included below.

Guidelines for Testing Hypotheses

1) The Behavior's Function Is to Escape Demands

Place demands on the individual. You may choose to ask her to perform many difficult academic tasks, or you may ask her to perform too-easy, boring tasks, depending on your hypothesis. You may want to place household demands on her, such as cleaning up toys, or you may choose to place social demands on her. Again, the demands you select will depend upon your hypotheses.

The child must be dealing with demands throughout the observation period. Therefore, choose tasks that have many steps and that will not be completed before the end of the observation period. For example, at home engage the child in: straightening out a room, a discrete trial session, or folding laundry. At school, engage her in: following an activity schedule, cleaning up a cubby, or completing a multi-step classwork assignment.

Try to provide as much attention as possible during the task. This way, you can control for an EO based on deprivation of general attention. One way to accomplish this is to provide instructions, redirection, and praise for completing the task. Additionally, use whatever other reinforcers you usually use for compliance. If the typical reinforcer takes time to enjoy and therefore would be time that the child is off task, stop timing the observation period and restart your timer when the reinforcement period ends. Similarly, use whatever consequence for problem behaviors that you typically use. If this takes an extended period of time (e.g., time out), then stop the timer as you would for a reinforcer. If your consequence for behaviors that occur during demand situations involve escape from demands, make a mental note of that. If your typical consequence does not involve allowing the child to escape from demands (e.g., redirecting her back to cleaning her room if she has a tantrum while cleaning it), then there is no need to stop and restart the timer.

2) The Behavior's Function Is to Obtain Attention

Give the child a couple of minutes of high-quality attention and then announce that you have something else to do (e.g., read a book, check your email, talk on the phone, etc.). Physically turn yourself away from her and do something else. Do not provide reinforcement in the form of attention throughout the observation period.

The person who is observing and recording the data should do so as covertly as possible. Try to watch out of the corner of your eye or to immediately look away if the child sees you watching her. If there is a window or television on in the room, you might try to position yourself so that it appears that you are looking out the window or watching television when you can, in fact, see the child from that angle.

Respond to any challenging behaviors as you normally would, being sure to stop the timer and restart it later if your response to a challenging behavior involves any attention. Remember, any attention is attention. This includes eye contact, yelling at the child, giving her a stern look, talking to her, patting her on the back, physically prompting her to an activity, etc.

Be sure that during this observation there are no demands on the child and that she has access to many preferred objects and activities. This allows you to control for other motivations to some degree.

3) The Behavior's Function Is to Get Access to Objects or Activities

Allow the child access to a number of preferred objects or activities. As she becomes interested in one, take it away. If possible, leave it where she can see it, but out of her reach. Announce that it is out of batteries, or too noisy, or that for some reason you want to save it for later. All the while that the desired item is out of reach, provide a rich level of attention and no demands. This will control for other motivations to some degree.

While some children—with and without an ASD—will wait patiently for the item and instead find another item or engage in some social interaction, other children will launch into a problem behavior to try to get the toy. If a child uses a problem behavior as a means of accessing preferred objects and activities, you can expect to see her display the problem behavior in an attempt to get the removed item back.

As with all of the experimental conditions, only the targeted behavior is counted, though you may wish to make note of other behaviors that occur.

4) The Behavior's Function Is Automatic Reinforcement

If a behavior is automatically reinforcing, then the person is not trying to give anyone a message through her behavior. Therefore, she may frequently engage in it when she is alone and does not have other things to do. Either use a video camera or stand outside the room and try to watch the child without being seen. Make sure she does not have any objects or activities nearby to fill her time. Do not enter the room or allow yourself to be seen unless it is necessary to preserve safety. This assessment is not appropriate for children with very dangerous behavior problems, for very young children, or for others who would not ordinarily be left alone in a room.

The key is to leave the child with nothing really to do, and see how she entertains herself. Some children might hum or sing songs, and others might engage in the challenging behavior. To make this condition less artificial, you can introduce it to the child as a "waiting" condition. Let the child know that you are going to go get something and that you'll be right back. This type of condition may elicit behaviors that occur as a result of the child being "bored."

An alternative to an "alone" condition is to look at the child's behavior during the control condition. Although you might miss the behaviors that occur as a result of boredom, if a problem behavior occurs when the child has access to all of the external stimuli she enjoys, then the only motivation to engage in the behavior would be to access internal stimuli.

Once your conditions are set, you can use the data sheet that matches the type of data you are collecting for your raw data and transfer totals to the Antecedent Manipulations Data Sheet found in Appendix I to allow for a clear comparison.

Using Cues to Signal Conditions

Each hypothesis-testing condition should be associated with a certain cue, if possible. This may help the child recognize the condition during subsequent testing sessions so that she will possibly engage in the problem behaviors more quickly. Cues you might consider include running different conditions in different rooms, draping different brightly colored towels over the couch for different sessions, or having the child sit in a different part of a room in different conditions. For example, if you are only comparing two conditions, you might leave the drapes open during one condition and closed during another. If your child is not happy with the arrangement (for example, asks to open drapes that are closed), you'll have to grant her request. Otherwise, you will create an unintentional restricted access condition (e.g., restricted access to looking out of the window).

If your child asks why the unusual item is placed where it is or the way it is, you can try to link it to whatever condition you are contriving. If you are about to do a low attention condition, for example, you can say that you've thrown a blanket over the couch because you are going to snuggle up in it while you read a book. If you are about to do a restricted access condition, you can explain that your put the blanket there so that you can keep her toy on it while it waits for new batteries.

Taking Safety Precautions

A special concern to think through before using antecedent manipulations is that you are essentially trying to elicit the problem behavior. Figuring out how you elicited it will let you know the behavior's function. However, for severe or dangerous behaviors, you must determine whether or not the benefits of conducting the assessment outweigh the risks of the behavior itself. For example, in the case of the head-banging student described above, if the student had not attended school in a highly specialized, resource-rich setting, it might have made sense to treat both possible functions of his behavior rather than run the risk that he might injure himself forcefully banging his head.

Always have a safety plan in case a behavior escalates under these conditions. You may want to have a safe place to direct the child to where she cannot hurt herself and can calm down. You may also want to have known distractors available if you need to end the assessment early. Protective gear, such as arm-pads or helmets, may be needed to prevent injury if a behavior escalates. It may also be wise to try to complete the assessment at a time when no other children are around. Finally, you may want a team member who is capable of physical restraint to be present.

Many individuals with autism spectrum disorders do not have extensive exposure to the conditions that elicit their behavior in everyday life because as soon as they engage in the behavior, people in their environment take steps to get them to stop before anyone is hurt. They may get a small dose of the eliciting condition, begin the prob-

---

Using the Antecedent Manipulation Strategy in School

The antecedent manipulation strategy can be introduced in any setting. In your home, or when working one on one with an individual in a classroom, it should be clear that you can simply set up the conditions as described above.

In a classroom setting, however, people often struggle with how to implement antecedent manipulation. For a model illustration of how to accomplish this, consider the work of Michael Mueller, Heather Sterling-Turner, and Dorothy Scattone. In 2001, these researchers published a study in the *Journal of Applied Behavior Analysis* describing their assessment of hand flapping by a typically developing five-year-old in a general education classroom. To summarize their approach, they developed a hypothesis through structured observation that the student flapped his hands when the task demands were too low. They instructed the teacher to conduct fifteen minutes of instruction with a low rate of demands, followed by fifteen minutes with a high rate of demands (on a schedule cued by the researchers). This sequence was then repeated. They measured hand flapping in each of the conditions and demonstrated that as the rate of demands went up, the rate of hand flapping went down. This led to a fairly simple intervention to help this student. Importantly, the assessment was conducted in a controlled, scientific fashion without disrupting the classroom, drawing attention to the student, or overwhelming the teacher.

lem behavior, and the condition ends. Because the goal of antecedent manipulation is a certain period of time under these conditions, the condition is continually reintroduced until the goal time is met. This might involve a greater degree of exposure to these conditions than the individual is used to. As a consequence, she may exhibit the behavior problem to a more intense degree. Keep this risk in mind as you decide whether or not to use the antecedent manipulation strategy.

After you have completed one round of antecedent manipulations, you should optimally repeat these conditions one or two more times to ensure that consistent patterns emerge. You should also prioritize safety when deciding how many replications of your assessment are possible.

Functional Analysis

As the term "antecedent manipulation" implies, only the antecedents are manipulated. In contrast, when conducting a functional analysis, both antecedents and consequences are controlled. To conduct a functional analysis, you set up specific environmental conditions, as with the antecedent manipulation strategy. Then, when a behavior occurs, instead of responding in your typical manner, you deliberately attempt to reinforce the problem behavior. In other words, when the problem behavior occurs, you give the child what you think she wants, reversing the antecedent conditions. For example, if the hypothesis is that your child is biting her teacher because she wants her attention, the teacher should provide attention when your child bites her.

For specific guidelines, see the chart on the next page which lists antecedents and consequences for the most common functional analysis conditions.

Why Is Functional Analysis Worthwhile?

You might wonder how any good at all can come of reinforcing a problem behavior. First, as discussed in our review of the research of

**Antecedents and Consequences for
Common Functional Analysis Conditions**

Antecedent Condition	Consequence for Problem Behavior
Low attention	Provide attention
Restricted access to preferred objects and activities	Provide access to objects and activities
High level of demands	Allow escape from demands
Control condition (used for comparison)	Ignore the behavior (continue attending to the individual)

Brian Iwata and his colleagues (1994), reinforcing a behavior gives us an opportunity to reenact what is happening in the child's everyday life. We can see which consequence has the power to strengthen the behavior within sessions. This gives us a good idea of what consequences are strengthening the behavior outside of sessions.

Some people voice concerns that a functional analysis will teach an individual that her inappropriate behavior is an effective method of communication and that she will have to "unlearn" this after the assessment process. Counter-intuitively, exposing someone with an ASD to a functional analysis might actually help her to unlearn a behavior more quickly. In everyday life, problem behaviors are usually reinforced inconsistently. The child never knows which instance of her behavior will be reinforced. Therefore, if at first she doesn't succeed, she keeps trying. Like a gambler playing a slot machine, she learns to persist in the behavior.

In contrast, during the assessment process, the individual with autism is getting reinforced for each instance of the behavior. This continual pattern of reinforcement actually teaches people to be less persistent. For example, every time you pick up your telephone, there is a dial tone. You are continually reinforced for picking up your phone. If there suddenly is no dial tone, after a brief bout of trying to identify the problem, you will give up and declare the phone dead. This is what we want to happen to our child with challenging behavior. If we take a behavior out of the intermittent reinforcement schedule that it receives in everyday life, and place it on the continuous schedule that it receives during a functional analysis, then the behavior may actually persist for less time during intervention.

Functional analyses are the gold standard of functional assessment. Results of a functional analysis are typically considered to be the most valid of any assessment tool. Volumes of research attest to the effectiveness of functional analysis in finding the communicative message of the behavior and in leading to successful interventions. However, they are labor intensive and involve certain risks (see below). Consequently, it may be best to reserve this strategy for exceptionally confusing behaviors for which other assessment approaches have failed. Additionally, because this approach involves eliciting and temporarily strengthening the problem behavior, it is best if only experienced professionals conduct functional analyses for very severe or dangerous behaviors. Furthermore, they should conduct their analyses in highly controlled settings.

There are inpatient placements available where functional analyses of even the most severe behavior problems can be implemented by teams of experts with the training and resources to preserve the safety of the child and themselves. If you are faced with a problem behavior that is extremely dangerous or destructive, or that has been unsuccessfully addressed by a skilled behavior analyst on an outpatient basis, consider an inpatient placement. The length of stay can vary widely from a few weeks to several months depending on how long it takes to identify distinct patterns of the behavior under different conditions. To find a local setting that can provide this type of service, check the Behavior Analyst Certification Board's website (www.bacb.com) and contact a local board-certified practitioner. He or she should be able to direct you to an appropriate provider.

Conducting a Functional Analysis

As with antecedent manipulation, you will begin by setting up your team, identifying the length of the session, and deciding which conditions to implement. Plan to implement a control condition along with any conditions needed to test specific hypotheses. Again, it is best for two people to be involved, one to interact with the child and one to observe and record data. However, as this may not always be possible, consider strategies described above for implementing the functional analysis alone.

Again as with antecedent manipulation, each session should introduce the antecedent condition for the same period of time and a specific cue should be associated with each condition. When a challenging behavior occurs, immediately provide the proposed reinforcer for a set amount of time. For a ten-minute session, thirty seconds of access to the reinforcer should be sufficient. For example, if your hypothesis is that your child is doing the behavior because she wants the TV on, you would switch it on for thirty seconds and then off again. While this might infuriate anyone, not everyone would display the specific problem behavior under study as a result. You might go a little higher or lower than thirty seconds in different circumstances depending on the unique patterns shown by the child. Just be sure that the time you use is consistent across sessions.

During a functional analysis, you are literally teaching the child to exhibit the behavior. To document this learning, you need to identify differences in the behavior under different conditions and to see patterns across time. For example, you may see that the frequency of head-hitting is increasing every session that the child is reinforced with a break from a challenging task, and staying low in all other conditions. This increase in behavior that you see indicates that learning has taken place and that the likely function of the behavior is escape.

Because you are looking for patterns, you will need to see multiple sessions of a functional analysis (unlike an antecedent manipulation where you replicate sessions only one or two times). Furthermore, graphing the information you collect will be critical here. Visually analyzing the data will help you to identify the function of the problem behavior. Always graph the data that you collect, in every condition.

Below is an example of a graph of a functional analysis. You can interpret the graph by looking at which condition led to the highest level of the behavior. Our sample graph suggests that the behavior being studied is likely to be maintained by escaping from demands. You can tell this because the behavior is most likely to occur during a high rate of demands, even during the first round of each session, and then continues to increase, which suggests that the consequence of escaping demands is strengthening it. As you can see, graphing functional analysis data is essential to interpreting it effectively.

Sample functional analysis data

Brief Functional Analyses

In some cases, the extended period of time needed to document learning through a functional analysis will not be feasible. Due to staffing constraints or the urgency of the intervention needed, a quicker experimental assessment is required. In these situations, consider conducting a brief functional analysis (Derby, Wacker, Sasso, Steege, Northup, Cigrand, & Asmus, 1992). A brief functional analysis is an adapted version of an extended functional analysis. Although researchers have described several variations on brief functional analysis methods, the classic design is intended to last no longer than ninety minutes.

In the first phase of a brief functional analysis, all possible functions of the target behavior are each tested once, as they would be during a standard functional analysis. For example, to evaluate

Grace's hitting, described in the Introduction, you would first run each of the four classic conditions as you would during a standard functional analysis: Escape, Attention, Restricted Access, and Automatic Reinforcement/Control.

Next, choose the conditions that elicited the highest and lowest rates of the target behavior. Let's imagine that for Grace, the highest was low attention and the lowest was escape. You would repeat just those two conditions. If the contrast in responding does not persist, you would need to back up and reevaluate other functions. However, if the pattern remains consistent, then a third phase is introduced. In this phase, team members cease reinforcing the target behavior and instead reinforce an appropriate functional alternative behavior. For Grace, they might ignore aggression and instead prompt and reinforce social greetings. The rates of both appropriate and inappropriate responses are measured to confirm that the correct function has been identified. Consider the following example:

Dana is a thirty-year-old woman with autism and mental retardation who has recently moved into a group home. She communicates only with gestures. Staff members are concerned because she has been biting her hand hard enough to cause significant damage. To use a brief functional analysis, the team assesses the hand biting under four conditions: Escape, Attention, Access, and Automatic Reinforcement/Control. Dana bites her hand the most in the access condition (specifically, when no cookies are available) and the least in the attention condition. Just these two conditions are then repeated. The results of these conditions mirror those that were originally obtained; restricted access to cookies elicits much higher rates of biting than does low attention.

At this point, the team has enough data to see that Dana consistently and frequently bites her hand when her access to cookies is restricted. They therefore decide to teach Dana a replacement skill (pointing) to help her request the restricted item (cookies) appropriately. The pattern of behavior now changes. Dana begins pointing at a high rate and virtually stops biting her hand. The data the team collected are shown on the chart on the next page.

Session Number	Condition	Number of bites	Number of points
1	Restricted access to cookies	12	1
2	Low attention	2	0
3	Restricted access	14	0
4	Reinforce pointing with cookies	3	10
5	Reinforce pointing with attention	2	2
6	Reinforce pointing with cookies	1	14

The following is another example of a brief functional analysis, but in this example, the assessment must take place in a preschool setting:

Daisy is a three-year-old girl with PDD-NOS who screams in school. This disturbing behavior interferes with Daisy's learning as well as that of her classmates. In order to complete a brief functional analysis of this behavior, Daisy's teacher, Heather, sets up four experimental conditions. Because Daisy is so young, Heather decides to make each session only five minutes long.

In the first session, Heather sets up a control condition by giving the class a five-minute snack break during which Daisy's favorite assistant teacher keeps her company. Next, for five minutes, Heather quizzes the class on colors and numbers, ensuring that Daisy is asked a question at least every minute. After that is completed, Heather sends Daisy to the reading corner with her favorite assistant teacher and has the assistant play and chat with Daisy for one minute before informing her that she has work to do so that Daisy will need to read and play by herself for a little while (five minutes). Finally, during the group craft that day, Heather tells Daisy that she will need to wait her turn for the glue (which is needed to complete a preferred project) and has her wait the entire five minutes.

For all of the above conditions, screaming is reinforced with a brief dose of the withheld motivator (e.g., screaming leads to a quick, maybe ten-second turn with the glue). Heather discovers that Daisy is the most likely to scream during low attention conditions and the least likely to scream during high demands. Next, she replicates only these two conditions. Again, screaming is most likely during low attention. Through prompting and reinforcement, Daisy is taught to say, "Let's talk" when she would like attention.

A five-minute low attention condition is now run during which Daisy's appropriate requests lead to attention but screaming does not. Daisy is also taught to request a break. A five-minute session of high demands is run during which both appropriate and inappropriate requests for breaks are unlikely. A final session of Daisy requesting attention is then run during which Daisy does not scream but makes frequent requests to play. Heather now feels confident that she has correctly identified the function of the behavior as being maintained by attention, and is well on her way to intervention.

8 | Putting It All Together
A Summary of the
Assessment Process

Reading through all of the strategies described in the preceding chapters can be overwhelming. You might be thinking, "Where do I begin?" The next page shows a flow chart that lists each of the steps in completing your functional behavior assessment.

After completing all of these steps, you should be able to use your findings to determine the function of the behavior. Following the description of each assessment tool included in this book, you will find directions as to how to use your data to identify the function of the behavior.

On the form starting on page 109, list the probable functions of the behavior you have come up with using each assessment tool.

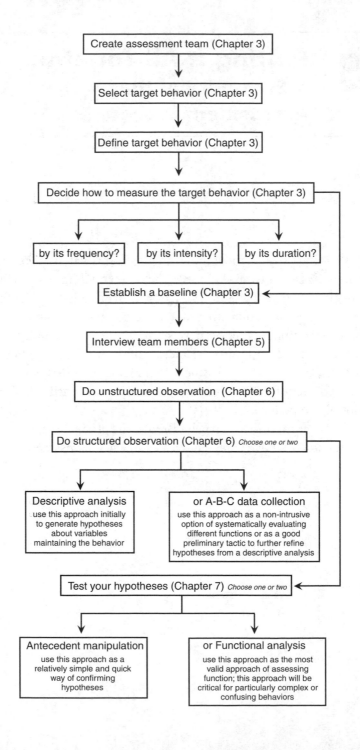

Functional Behavior Assessment Summary Form

Behavior: _____

Definition of Behavior:

_____

_____

_____

_____

Did you suspect any particular function(s) before completing the
assessment? If yes, please list:

1. _____
2. _____
3. _____

After reviewing interview data, what are the most likely function(s)?

1. _____
2. _____
3. _____

Based on unstructured observation, what are the most likely function(s)?

1. _____
2. _____
3. _____

Based on structured observation, what are the most likely function(s)?

1. _____
2. _____
3. _____

(Continued on next page.)

Based on hypothesis testing, what are the most likely function(s)?

1. _____

2. _____

3. _____

Any consistent predominant function(s)?

1. _____

2. _____

3. _____

Notes:

If inconsistent across all tools, does a consistent function emerge within each setting? If so, behavior probably serves a different function in each setting.

If inconsistent across all tools, and inconsistent across settings, behavior probably serves multiple functions in each setting.

9 | You Finally Know the Function of the Behavior: Now What?

Congratulations! All your hard work has paid off! You finally know why that seemingly senseless behavior keeps occurring. But, now what? How will this information help you? Detailed instruction regarding setting up a functionally relevant behavior plan is beyond the scope of this book. Nevertheless, because knowing how you will use your assessment information is critical in understanding the assessment process, an introduction to the development of behavior plans is included below. In the forthcoming companion volume to this book, I will cover this topic in much greater detail.

What Are the Components of an Intervention Plan?

Just as the assessment process grows out of what we know about learning, so does the intervention process. Remember those four keys to learning?
1. The establishing operation (EO),
2. the immediate antecedent,
3. the behavior, and
4. the consequence.

It turns out these are the keys to unlearning problem behaviors as well. Therefore, when creating functionally relevant behavior intervention plans, we focus on each of these critical variables. For every behavior plan, each of the four keys to learning must be considered.

Change the EO

First, to change a behavior, you can alter the child's EO for the behavior. If there is no EO for the behavior in place, it will not occur.

One way to alter the EO for a given behavior is to enrich the person's environment in such a way that the behavior will never be evoked. For example, if a child has a problem behavior in order to obtain attention, then provide a greater degree of attention throughout the day. Specifically, if you know that she usually lasts about ten minutes without attention before exhibiting the problem behavior, be sure to provide attention at least every eight minutes. Over time, other teaching strategies can be introduced to help her tolerate longer and longer periods of low attention. By controlling the establishing operation in this way, you can ensure that the target behavior never occurs. This will prevent the individual from practicing the behavior, which prevents her from being reinforced for the behavior, which ultimately helps make the behavior obsolete.

Some points of intervention that fall under this approach include:

1. addressing any issues related to physiological problems (e.g., a child who uses problem behaviors to escape a task because she is too sleepy to work, or a child whose allergies make her too uncomfortable to concentrate on a social interaction);
2. setting-related variables (e.g., a child who uses a behavior to escape a too brightly lit environment, or an adolescent who engages in self-talk whenever things are too quiet); or
3. contextual variables (e.g., a child who exhibits behavior problems in crowds, or an adult who has behavior problems only when she is assigned housekeeping duties at the hotel where she works.)

In many cases, addressing the behavior from this standpoint alone will eliminate a problem behavior. The downside of using this approach in isolation is that the individual does not learn how to manage that EO if it arises in some less-controlled setting. Because it is often impossible to prevent a specific EO from ever being in effect, it is almost guaranteed that the person will need to learn the skill of managing that EO effectively.

Change the Antecedents

Next, an intervention focuses on immediate antecedents. If consistent immediate antecedents have been identified through your assessment, you will want to examine these and attempt to change them where possible. Sometimes changing a seemingly minor cue will completely alter a behavior. For example, if a child exhibits challenging behaviors whenever she sees her work desk, allowing her to work on the floor instead can help to eliminate the behavior. Similarly, if a child has a history of resisting bedtime, she may be more cooperative if you call it "rest time."

Of course, you cannot always rely on this approach. When potty training, for example, the toilet will always be involved. If sirens set off a behavior, you cannot shield the student from sirens forever. Furthermore, changing antecedents may not be an option for automatic reinforcement behaviors, as the antecedent may sometimes occur inside of the person.

Change the Behavior

The third key component in the learning equation is the behavior itself. In your intervention plan, you will not only attempt to rid the individual of the problem behavior, but you will also ensure that she acquires a new behavior to get her needs met.

This step is probably the most critical in developing a successful plan. You will want to choose a replacement behavior that is simple for the individual to acquire and will lead to reinforcement for her. Recall from our overview of learning theory that a more efficient behavior will always replace a less efficient behavior. Therefore, replacement behaviors must be carefully selected to compete with problem behaviors. You need to find a behavior that will allow her to get what she wants more quickly and consistently than the problem behavior does. For example, if Kayla vomits after taking one bite of food as a way of avoiding eating certain meals, we can teach her to ask for something different. If Joey hits the teacher when the work is too boring, we can teach him to ask for different work.

Similarly, if Anthony is banging his head as a means of requesting his favorite beads, then you might teach him to hand over a picture card to request the beads. This would be an effective replacement behavior only if the card is clearly identifiable, easily accessible, and entails minimal challenge for Anthony. In short, the picture exchange will replace the head banging if it is an easier way to obtain the same result.

In order to teach Anthony to request the beads using the picture exchange, you might consider hanging a photo of the beads in every room. Starting in one room with the beads next to you but out of his reach, you might prompt Anthony to take the card and hand it to you. Then, you'd say something like, "Oh, you want the beads; great telling me you want the beads," as you hand him the beads. After two or three minutes with the beads, you would remove the beads, again placing them within his sight, but out of his reach. The entire process would then be repeated. After a few cycles fully prompted, you might gradually fade back your prompts and see if Anthony can request the beads independently in this scenario. As he gains proficiency at this, you would gradually increase the demand by increasing Anthony's distance from the beads, and gradually putting them out of sight. Once Anthony was proficient at requesting the beads with the photo when he was in the room with them, you would have him practice in other rooms. At that point, Anthony should start to request the beads independently.

In some cases, it might take an individual quite a while to learn a replacement skill, but teaching the replacement skill should nevertheless be part of the intervention, as this will be critical in maintaining long-term success.

Change the Consequences

The final component in the learning equation is the consequence. When intervening on a problem behavior, you will aim to reverse the consequence that has historically been typical. Continuing our above example, Anthony must no longer get the beads as a consequence for head banging. Instead, Anthony should receive beads immediately for using his picture exchange.

Sometimes it will not be possible to immediately reverse the consequence of a problem behavior. This is more likely to be the case if self-injurious or otherwise dangerous behavior is involved. Perhaps Anthony's family needs to give Anthony the beads to get him to stop banging his head. In cases like this, be sure that the consequence for the replacement behavior far surpasses the consequence for the challenging behavior in terms of quality and quantity. This contrast will lead the challenging behavior to disappear. Based on this principle, Anthony's family might give Anthony two or three of the least interesting beads if he bangs his head, but twenty or thirty of his favorite beads if he requests beads with his picture card.

When a child is more verbal or has stronger cognitive skills, it might be helpful to let her know about the change in rules and consequences. For example, Darra's mother, from our introduction, might say something to her like, "Darra, I know you love to talk about Clay Aiken, but other people get tired of hearing about him all day. Other kids would probably be more interested in being your friend if you sometimes talked about things *they* wanted to talk about. I'm afraid I'm going to have to ignore you if you talk about Clay, but I will be happy to talk with you about anything else...."

As with any behavioral intervention, informing someone of the new rules means nothing if you don't stick to what you say. Therefore, before reversing any contingency, be sure to choose an approach that you, and everyone else responsible for working with your child, can stick to. For example, if Darra's mother knows that Darra's teacher gets so irritated by the Clay Aiken talk that she will not be able to ignore it, then another approach that everyone can consistently use must be selected.

Choosing Strategies to Match the Function of the Behavior

The guidelines described above highlight the various components of an intervention. Next, you will learn some basic/beginning steps to developing each of these components for a specific behavior based on your functional behavior assessment results. To accomplish this, further assessment questions remain. The answers to these questions will help pinpoint specific strategies. Further assessment questions for the four basic functions of behavior are included below:

For Attention-Maintained Behaviors

What is the quality of attention that the person with an ASD is seeking?

- Will any attention do?
- Is it peer attention?
- Is it adult attention?
- Is it undivided attention?
- Is it high intensity attention?
- Is it physical attention?
- Is it a certain person's attention?
- How long can the child go between instances of this type of attention without exhibiting the problem behavior?

Use the answers to these questions to guide your intervention. For example, if your child uses her problem behavior to get high intensity attention, you should give her that attention on a rich schedule regardless of her behavior. Additionally, you should praise her in an animated and high intensity fashion. Furthermore, you might teach her to request a game that results in high intensity attention (e.g., tickle tag) and reinforce these requests consistently at first. Problem behaviors should not result in obtaining the desired attention.

Although you cannot consistently control all of the variables, such as peer attention, you will be surprised at how much you can actually accomplish by putting forth your best effort. For example, if a child is using a problem behavior (e.g., wisecracks) to get his classmates' attention, setting up class-wide contingencies (such as establishing a rule that anyone who laughs at another student's wisecracks during class gets five extra minutes of homework) can cut peer attention enough to make the intervention effective.

For Escape-Maintained Behaviors

- What is the individual with autism escaping?
- Is the demand too challenging?
- Is the demand too boring?
- Is the demand centered around non-preferred materials?
- Is the demand associated with a certain type of stimulation?
- Is the demand social?
- Is the demand specific to a certain person?
- Does the demand go on for too long?

Again, you will create your intervention around the answers to these questions. For example, a behavior that occurs because a task is too boring might be addressed by making the task a bit harder, using more preferred materials, and tackling goals in a more preferred format (e.g., playing a game rather than completing a worksheet). You might teach your child to appropriately request new tasks and consistently reinforce appropriate requests at first. Problem behaviors should not result in escaping the demand.

In some cases, a behavior might be reinforced by removing a stimulus or a person that you do not want removed. For example, one child might exhibit a problem behavior to escape or avoid taking a bath. However, you cannot just teach your child to request to skip her bath, as she needs to be clean. In this instance, you might try to isolate the variable that is aversive to your child. For example, does she especially dislike the water running in her face during shampooing? Then, having her wear a visor might solve the problem. Does she dislike the washcloth? Try using a scrubbing puff.

Similarly, a child's sometimes uses a problem behavior to avoid contact with certain people, such as a sibling or a specific instructor. Nevertheless, escaping these people permanently is not an option. For this situation, use the same approach used in our bath example above. Try to identify what it is about the person that the child finds aversive. Is the sibling's presence associated with less attention from Mom? Then perhaps you should really be intervening based on divided attention. Is the sibling associated with any positive activities? If not, perhaps pairing the sibling with the child's favorite treats and activities will help. Sometimes some idiosyncratic variable is responsible for avoidance of certain individuals, like the smell of someone's perfume or the sound of their squeaky sneakers. Once identified, these variables are simple to address.

For Behaviors Maintained By Access to Objects and Activities

- What activities or objects does the individual get from the behavior?
- Does the behavior occur when it's time to give up access?
- Does the behavior occur when she needs to wait for access?
- Does the behavior occur when she needs to share?
- Does the behavior occur when she needs to take turns?

As with the behavior plan ideas listed above, you will create your intervention around the answers to these questions. For example, a behavior that occurs when a child needs to take turns might be addressed by giving her more access to the item throughout the day, offering warnings of how much time is left before she needs to give up her turn, teaching her to request a little more time and initially reinforcing this request, providing a powerful reinforcer for sharing, and requiring her to share even if she exhibits the problem behavior.

For Behaviors Maintained by Automatic Reinforcement

- What exactly is the sensation that the individual is obtaining with the problem behavior?
- Is the behavior related to a medical problem (e.g., head banging during an ear infection)?

Automatic reinforcement behaviors are the trickiest to tackle. First of all, identifying the exact sensation that the child is obtaining from the problem behavior may pose a challenge. If possible, try the behavior yourself to see what sensations you experience. Some common sensations associated with automatic behaviors include vestibular stimulation (e.g., from rocking or spinning), dizziness, visual input (e.g., from watching hand-flapping or running back and forth by a fence), feeling pleasurable textures (e.g., from rubbing stockings or handling soft materials), a meditative state (e.g., from humming or rocking), or reliving pleasurable experiences (e.g., from self-talk or singing).

People often wonder what type of desirable feedback could possibly come from self-injury. One plausible theory suggests that endorphins, chemicals associated with peaceful and happy feelings that are naturally released in the brain in response to an injury, are somehow more acutely active for these individuals than for the average person. If that were indeed the case, then it would make sense that self-injury would lead to a sense of "rush."

If you cannot try the behavior yourself, as in the case of self-injurious or dangerous behaviors, you will have to use trial and error to try to determine what the person gets out of the behavior. Obviously, if the behavior is related to a medical problem, treat the medical problem.

Once you have an idea of the sensation the individual is getting from her behavior, try to identify a more appropriate source of the same stimulation for her. Some common examples might involve introducing a rocking chair for someone who rocks, a portable CD player for someone who sings to herself, a fan for someone who flaps her hands, or gloves for someone who wraps her own hands up with fabric.

You can also try to link the behavior to a certain setting. For example, you might try to establish a "talking chair," or a chair that serves as the only place a child is allowed to engage in self-talk. Then, any time you observe your child talking to herself, you would guide her to that chair. This approach can also work for people who need others around to satisfy their motivation. For example, if Darra wants to talk to someone about Clay, you could designate one specific person who will listen to the talk in one specific place. For example, Darra could talk to her mom in her room. If she started to talk about Clay at school, her teachers could interrupt and tell her that discussing Clay is something special between her and her mother. At home, Darra could be taught to say to her mother, "Can we go to my room and talk about Clay?" A timer could then be set and she could have her need met without stigmatizing herself. As long as Clay talk is not responded to or accepted in other environments or with other people, Darra would quickly learn to make this request.

In our everyday lives, we learn contingencies such as this all the time. For example, we all have friends who gossip, and friends who don't. We have friends to whom we admit that we ate an entire box of cookies, and friends who would be disgusted by that. We quickly learn these contingencies and get our reinforcement where we can.

In general, effective intervention for automatic reinforcement behaviors focuses on finding a harmless way to get the child the stimulation that she is seeking. Like any other attempts to stop a behavior without teaching new skills, they will be fruitless if the child does not have another way to get her needs met.

One of the easiest strategies for targeting automatic reinforcement behaviors involves enriching the environment with preferred objects, people, and activities. Often if the child is provided with sufficient external stimulation, she no longer feels the need to stimulate herself.

10 | Special Circumstances and Troubleshooting

For assessing all but the most challenging behaviors in children and adults with autism spectrum disorders, the information and guidelines presented up until this point will be sufficient to lead to effective intervention. Nevertheless, there are some situations that require special attention for various reasons. For example, there are some special considerations to keep in mind when doing functional behavior assessments of adolescents or adults, or when assessing dangerous but infrequent behaviors. To meet these challenges, you'll need to become a functional behavior assessment "specialist." Ideas for working with these special populations and situations, as well as for troubleshooting when behavioral functions and interventions are not clear, are included below.

Adolescents and Adults

Although you will use the same general strategies for completing functional behavior assessments with adolescents and adults that you use with children, there are some special considerations to keep in mind.

Safety Issues

First and foremost, keep the individual's size in mind. Because adolescents and adults are bigger and stronger than younger children, you will need to exercise particular caution with regard to escalation of behaviors. As you would when completing an assessment with a child, be sure to stop any assessment that is placing someone in danger and switch to crisis management mode immediately. "Crisis management" mode implies that a long-term treatment for a behavior is no longer the priority. Instead, preserving everyone's safety becomes an immediate priority. This might translate into actually reinforcing a challenging behavior (assuming that you know what will do so) in order to make it end. While this is counterintuitive regarding the treatment of challenging behaviors, it is the logical choice in the realm of common sense—safety first! You can follow up with a thorough assessment and intervention later.

Some of the assessment strategies described actually elicit the problem behavior, and may even elicit a more intense form of the behavior. Do not use these approaches when assessing aggressive, self-injurious, or destructive behaviors without the supervision of an experienced behavior analyst trained in crisis management procedures. If such supervision is not available, consider inpatient placement at a facility where the function of the behavior can be identified while preserving everyone's safety. Contact your school district or a local board certified behavior analyst (see www.BACB.com) for assistance in finding an inpatient placement near you.

As a final safety note, when choosing interventions for adolescents and adults with potentially dangerous behaviors, consider relying on interventions based on changing EO's and immediate antecedents whenever possible. This will preserve safety for everyone, as it will prevent the behavior from occurring at all, rather than requiring attempts to respond to it.

Some clients I have worked with question whether or not it is acceptable for these proactive interventions to be in place permanently to prevent the problem behavior. They are concerned that the individual is not functioning independently if he always needs these supports. For example, consider a young man with autism and mental retardation who requires brief social attention such as a smile and pat on the back every fifteen minutes in order to prevent severe, destructive behaviors. Would I recommend that this intervention remain in place permanently? I absolutely would. Unless it would cause significant hardship to those around the individual, leaving an intervention in place permanently to avoid a serious behavior problem would be worth it.

Just as some individuals have disabilities that require wheelchairs, or the use of braille, some individuals have disabilities that require other forms of support. As long as it is feasible to provide what is needed, I would not be concerned about whether or not a person "should" need a support that prevents significant problem behaviors. Teaching the person to do without that support may be possible, but why not improve the quality of his life and skip all of the risk involved in trying to teach him to do without it at the same time?

Allowing Enough Time to Learn a New Behavior

Another consideration when addressing problem behaviors in adolescents and adults is the length of time they have engaged in the problem behavior. Depending on the particular behavior, the individual may have been effectively practicing a certain problematic response for a very long time. The longer a behavior has been practiced, the longer it will take to be replaced. For example, have you ever written the previous year on a check just after New Year's? It takes a while to unlearn the well-practiced response of writing the previous year. Have you ever moved to a new home and accidentally written your old return address on an envelope? You had practiced writing the previous address for a long time and it will take longer to stop that practice than it would to stop writing an address you've written once or twice. When a behavior has persisted a long time, it should be easier to elicit during the assessment process but take longer to successfully address during intervention.

On the flip side, do not assume that because adolescents and adults are older, they have had an opportunity to learn appropriate behaviors. When older adults with pervasive developmental disorders were children, teaching strategies were not as sophisticated as they are today. Every year, the field progresses and existing teaching practices may be improved. When completing a functional behavior assessment for an adolescent or adult, pay particularly close attention to assessing communication skills as well as to identifying what activities the person can perform independently. Also try to take note of how much access he has to his preferences. Especially if someone has a more limited educational history, you may find that others have very little knowledge of his preferences. Consequently, his life is probably desperately in need of enrichment.

Part of an assessment for someone in this situation might involve comparing the strength of the behavior under enriched versus impoverished environments. For example, imagine an adult who has lived in an institutional setting for most of his life who is now moving into a group home. This individual may at first exhibit many significant behavior problems. As group home staff become more familiar with this man, they may discover that he likes to take walks, or that he enjoys watching "Wheel of Fortune." They may also discover that his favorite food is waffles and his favorite drink is tea. They may teach him some requesting skills to obtain preferred items and activities. Furthermore, he might receive much more attention than he did in his institutional placement. In this new, enriched environment, it would be very surprising if we did not see his behavior problems decrease. As more of his needs are met, and he has more skills to get his needs met, there would be less and less reason for him to exhibit a challenging behavior.

Choosing the Right Setting for an Assessment

Finally, when working with adolescents and adults, you may need to assess behaviors that occur outside the home or school. For example, you may be faced with assessing a problem behavior that occurs on a job site. Eliciting the behavior in that setting may be frightening and confusing to customers or other workers who might be present. In this case, you might have to replicate the conditions on the job site as best as possible in a more controlled setting, such as the individual's classroom or home. This might involve role playing by members of the assessment team, or it might involve inviting people from the job site to come to the classroom or home.

For individuals who live in supervised settings such as a group home or institution, you may be faced with privacy concerns when completing your assessment. For example, other clients should not have access to information about one particular client's problem behavior or assessment conditions. Finding a place to conduct the assessment without the other residents' awareness might pose a challenge.

A particularly challenging situation could arise if an adult with ASD exhibits a behavior that disturbs a roommate or that elicits problem behaviors from a housemate. To the best of your ability, you must keep the housemate safe and communicate to him or her that the behavior is being addressed, without sharing any more information than is necessary.

Keep these variables in mind when conducting your assessment. Be sure to speak to relevant staff to gather necessary information.

Rare, but Dangerous, Behaviors

Some behaviors occur very infrequently, but nevertheless pose significant risks to people and property. The severity of these behaviors demands intervention, yet their low rate of occurrence prevents us from observing naturally occurring patterns in the behavior or from contriving situations to elicit the behavior. For instance, one adolescent with whom I worked had such severe aggressive behavior and tantrums on the bus ride home from school that the driver feared for his own safety and had to pull over and call school personnel to come and pick up the student. This happened twice throughout the entire school year. As you might imagine, it was very hard to gather information as to the function of the behavior since so little observational data was available.

For these types of behaviors, special assessment procedures are required. As with other behaviors, you will still assemble an intervention team, define the behavior, and determine how to measure it if it does occur. However, you may not be able to establish a baseline as you would with other behaviors because too much time might pass between occurrences for a pattern to be established. Rely heavily on interviewing people familiar with the individual and the behavior to gather as much information about patterns of the behavior as possible. Also, ask those who have observed the behavior to complete A-B-C data sheets from memory.

Although relying on recall of events is not ideal, consistent responses from multiple observers can support resulting hypotheses. Based on these information gathering approaches, you are poised to develop some ideas about the possible function of the behavior, institute an interim intervention, and to gather more information about the behavior if it does recur.

Finally, everyone who might be responsible for the individual at any given time must be provided with training in crisis management strategies to preserve everyone's safety. For the student who exhibited dangerous behaviors on the bus, interviews with those close to the child suggested that he was most likely to engage in problem behavior when he was receiving little attention and had nothing else to do. Consequently, he was provided with a bag of preferred snacks and activities for the bus ride, and the driver was trained to interact with him briefly every few minutes. This approach was effective in preventing further occurrences of the behavior.

Troubleshooting

There are two broad types of trouble spots that arise when using functional behavior assessment with people with autism spectrum disorders. They arise when:

1. The assessment results are highly inconsistent, making it difficult to determine the function of the behavior. Or:

2. You think you have determined the function of the behavior, but an intervention designed around that function does not work.

When Assessment Results Are Inconsistent

The first stumbling block that may arise is highly inconsistent assessment results. In this scenario, any or all of the following may be true:

- Each person interviewed by the team coordinator offers different information and different opinions about why the behavior is occurring.
- No two reporters agree on the actual antecedents and consequences of the behavior.
- Observational data yield inconsistent results.

Sometimes assessment results are inconsistent because the behavior is so unclear. Other times this might occur when different observers and reporters have preconceived notions about the behavior that they are seeking to affirm. In other circumstances, conflicting reports may result because reporters perceive pressure to paint a certain picture. For example, teaching staff may not want to suggest that the behavior occurs because their student's work is too uninteresting. Face these problems head on when you suspect them and reassure staff that your assessment is not an evaluation of their work.

Nevertheless, despite your best efforts, you might remain stumped. Try your best to assess just one variable at a time and be creative and observant in developing your hypotheses.

If you remain stumped after your best efforts, try an intervention that addresses attention, escape from demands, and access to preferred items. For example, you might teach a child appropriate requests for all three potential reinforcers, do your best not to respond at all to the challenging behavior when it occurs, and enrich the child's environment with attention, preferred items and activities, and interesting, functional tasks. This will likely lead to decreases in the problem behavior, although you may never find out why.

When an Intervention Doesn't Work

A second stumbling block that may occur relates to the intervention. You have completed a thorough functional behavior assessment and you are sure that you have identified the function of the behavior. You develop an intervention based on these findings and—it doesn't work. First, there are various aspects of the intervention to evaluate:

- Does it actually match the function identified?
- Does it address EO's, antecedents, replacement behaviors, and consequences?
- Is it being implemented according to plan? By everyone who encounters the behavior?

If the answer to all of these questions is yes, you may need to complete a brief reassessment of the behavior. It is possible for the function of a behavior to change. For example, one child I worked with used to spit during teaching sessions because he enjoyed watching the spit fly through the air and land on something. Part of the intervention that was developed for this behavior involved having him wipe up the spit immediately. Because this intervention was implemented during teaching sessions, it often delayed his work so that he would get less work done each day. This student quickly learned to use the spitting behavior to meet a second function of escaping class work. A new plan addressing escape from task in addition to automatic reinforcement needed to be developed. This plan involved reworking the student's tasks to make them more appropriate and interesting, teaching him an appropriate way to request a break, and ignoring the spitting, as well as allowing him to request to spit into the toilet.

If you need to reassess a behavior after a plan has been developed, a briefer assessment may suffice. First, the behavior will already be defined and a measurement system will already be developed. Consider relying on just a couple of interviews as well as some structured observation. This abbreviated approach coupled with careful thinking about how the plan changed the environment for the child may lead to a successful intervention.

Some behaviors may take a little longer to change. Recall that the longer a behavior is in a child's repertoire, the longer it will take to change. These behaviors will eventually be replaced as the child practices replacement behaviors and receives reinforcement for them. Returning to our example about writing the correct year on checks, we all eventually do learn to write the correct year. Similarly, if you drive "on autopilot" and keep finding yourself heading to your old home after you have moved, you will eventually start driving to your new home. Challenging behaviors are no different; these too will eventually be replaced.

Some behaviors based on avoidance may be particularly difficult to change. Each time the feared scenario is avoided, the escape behavior grows stronger. Imagine Lily, a three-year-old girl who develops a painful urinary tract infection and then refuses to urinate. She has to be taken to the hospital and catheterized and after this harrowing experience still refuses to urinate. Each time she avoids urination and her perception of the associated pain, her avoidance behaviors are strengthened. Because she experienced the pain associated with urination on an intermittent schedule, urinating once or twice without pain does not convince her that it will be painless the next time.

For avoidance behaviors of this nature, consider a number of strategies. First, if possible, teach the child how to respond if the feared event does occur. For instance, Lily could be reminded that she can stop urination in midstream and any pain will stop instantly. Also consider using strong motivators for completing the behavior. For Lily, a star chart leading to ice cream (a highly preferred consequence) actually worked in getting her to resume urination. Finally, consider changing the environment where the avoided activity or item is encountered. For Lily, you might try a different bathroom than she usually uses, introduce a potty seat on top of the toilet, mildly redecorate the bathroom with new character towels and pictures, or let her decorate the lid of the toilet with removable stickers.

Success Stories

Aaron

Aaron was a fifteen-year-old boy with PDD-NOS. Aaron's favorite way to interact with people was to poke, swat, and tickle them. Aaron poked his peers, his teachers, his parents, his siblings, and familiar adults who came over to the house. Because Aaron was in an inclusive educational setting, this behavior was extremely stigmatizing for him. During participation in a mainstream camp setting, Aaron had unfortunately been severely teased by the boys in his group as a result of the poking. Although he was devastated by their treatment of him, he persisted in poking.

Interview and observation left some confusion about whether the behavior was maintained by attention or based on automatic reinforcement. Through antecedent manipulations, it was determined that the behavior primarily served an automatic reinforcement function, although some team members argued vehemently that attention-seeking played a role. The team members agreed that the automatic reinforcement function would be treated first, and they could see how much of the behavior was left, and in which settings it occurred.

Treatment involved teaching Aaron to request "tickle time" and also offering it to him at least once each day. "Tickle time" initially took place in the playroom with Aaron's mother only, but was later transferred to Aaron's one-to-one instructor when the level of touch became uncomfortable for Aaron's mother. Whenever Aaron initiated poking outside of "tickle time," he was reminded that there was a specific time and place where that occurred. During "tickle time," Aaron and his instructor poked, swatted, and tickled intensely and laughed and thoroughly enjoyed themselves. By the end of the school year, Aaron's poking behavior had disappeared entirely from all settings except during the designated tickle time. In fact, there never was a need to address any supposed attention issues related to the behavior.

Sophie

Sophie was a five-year-old girl who loved other children but lacked the social skills to initiate interactions with them effectively. In a group, Sophie used to immediately run up to other children and provoke them while laughing and smiling. She might push them, steal their toys, or pull their hair. Interview and structured observation strongly agreed that Sophie used these behaviors in order to obtain attention from *peers. It was decided that there was enough confidence based on these two assessment techniques that no further assessment was needed.*

In order to treat Sophie's rough and tumble initiation strategy, she was provided with scripted language to use with peers just prior to each play date or group socialization activity. In particular, three comments or questions that Sophie could use with peers were modeled for her each time. Additionally, Sophie was promised ten minutes of extra playtime for keeping her hands to herself throughout the interaction. Data collection included measuring Sophie's physical behaviors as well as whether or not she used one of the modeled phrases. Almost immediately, Sophie replaced her more aggressive methods with these newly modeled phrases. After two months, Sophie began generalizing previously modeled phrases and coming up with original conversation openers of her own. Finally, the modeling was dropped and Sophie continued to keep her hands off the other children. The naturally occurring reinforcement from peers for her more appropriate initiations was all the motivation that Sophie needed to maintain her newly acquired skills.

Ramone

Ramone was an eighteen-year-old man with autism who was admitted to a day program for individuals with severe behaviors. In particular, Ramone punched staff members, other clients, and visitors to the program. Interview and observation had revealed that punching was likely when there were crowds, during work tasks, during social demands, and when Ramone wanted food or drinks, but no specific predominant function had been identified. Furthermore, antecedent manipulations did not implicate one function as stronger than the others.

Because his behaviors were so severe, Ramone had historically been allowed to do whatever he liked, unfettered by demands or restrictions. In part because prior staff had hesitated to place educational demands upon him, Ramone had no communication system other than grunting and limited gesturing.

As a first step, Ramone's environment was enriched through a "pairing" procedure in which an attempt was made to associate staff and the new setting with preferred items and activities. Ramone was given plenty of free access to preferred items and activities. Next, Ramone was taught a few basic communicative signs. In particular, he was taught to request certain food items, to request some space, to request a break, and to request attention. Finally, whenever he punched, he continued to be restrained, as staff feared for their safety. These simple changes led to a huge decrease in Ramone's aggressive behavior. This decrease was maintained across time and carried over into the home. Eventually, Ramone's aggression diminished so much that he was able to obtain supervised employment and work outside of the school.

References

Austin, J., Weatherly, N. L., & Gravina, N. E. (2005). Using task clarification, graphic feedback, and verbal feedback to increase closing-task completion in a privately owned restaurant. *Journal of Applied Behavior Analysis, 38,* 117-20.

Catania, A. C. (1998). *Learning.* Upper Saddle River, NJ: Simon & Schuster.

Delmolino, L. & Harris, S. (2004). *Incentives for Change: Motivating People with Autism Spectrum Disorders to Learn and Gain Independence.* Bethesda, MD: Woodbine House.

Durand, V. M. & Crimmins, D. B. (1988). Identifying variables maintaining self-injurious behavior. *Journal of Autism and Developmental Disabilities, 18,* 99-117.

Ervin, R. A., DuPaul, G. J., Kern, L., & Friman, P. C. (1998). Classroom-based functional and adjunctive assessments: Proactive approaches to intervention selection for adolescents with attention deficit hyperactivity disorder. *Journal of Applied Behavior Analysis, 31,* 65-78.

Ferster, C. B. (1958). Control of behavior in chimpanzees and pigeons by time out from positive reinforcement. *Psychological Monographs, 72,* 108.

Frea, W. D. & Hughes, C. (1997). Functional analysis and treatment of social-communicative behavior of adolescents with developmental disabilities. *Journal of Applied Behavior Analysis, 30,* 701-704.

Hanley, G. P., Piazza, C. C., Fisher, W. W., & Maglieri, K. A. (2005). On the effectiveness of and preference for punishment and extinction components of function-based interventions. *Journal of Applied Behavior Analysis, 38,* 51-65.

Individuals with Disabilities Education Act Amendments of 1997, 20 U.S.C. 1401-1485.

Iwata, B. A., Pace, G. M., Dorsey, M. F., Zarcone, J. R., Vollmer, T. R., Smith, R. G., Rodgers, T. A., Lerman, D. C., Shore, B. A., Mazaleski, J. L., Goh, H.-L., Cowdery, G. E., Kalsher, M. J., McCosh, K. C., & Willis, K. D. (1994). The functions of self-injurious behavior: An experimental-epidemiological analysis. *Journal of Applied Behavior Analysis, 27,* 215-40.

Iwata, B. A., Dorsey, M. F., Slifer, K. J., Bauman. K. E., & Richman, G. S. (1982). Toward a functional analysis of self-injury. *Analysis and Intervention in Developmental Disabilities, 2,* 3-20.

Kern, L., Dunlap, G., Clarke, S., & Childs, K. (1994). Student-assisted functional assessment interview. *Diagnostique, 19 (2-3),* 29-39.

Kwak, M. M., Ervin, R. A., Anderson, M. Z., & Austin, J. (2004). Agreement of function across methods used in school-based functional assessment with preadolescent and adolescent students. *Behavior Modification, 28 (3),* 375-401.

Michael, J. (1982). Distinguishing between discriminative and motivational functions of stimuli. *Journal of the Experimental Analysis of Behavior, 37,* 149-55.

Mueller, M. M., Sterling-Turner, H. E., & Scattone, D. (2001). Functional assessment of hand flapping in a general education classroom. *Journal of Applied Behavior Analysis, 34,* 233-36.

Ratner, S. C. (1970). Habituation: Research and theory. In J. H. Reynierse (Ed.), *Current issues in animal learning* (pp. 55-84). Lincoln, NE: University of Nebraska Press.

Reed, H., Thomas, E., Sprague, J. R. & Horner, R. H. (1997). The student guided functional assessment interview: An analysis of student and teacher agreement. *Journal of Behavioral Education, 7 (1),* 33-49.

Repp, A. C., Felce, D., & Barton, L. E. (1988). Basing the treatment of stereotypic and self-injurious behaviors on hypotheses of their causes. *Journal of Applied Behavior Analysis, 21,* 281-89.

Skinner, B. F. (1953). *Science and Human Behavior.* New York, NY: The Macmillan Company.

Skinner, B. F. (1984). The operational analysis of psychological terms. *Behavioral and Brain Sciences, 7,* 547-82.

Vollmer, T. R. & Iwata, B. A. (1991). Establishing operations and reinforcement effects. *Journal of Applied Behavior Analysis, 24,* 279-91.

Appendices

Appendix A
Frequency Recording Data Sheet

Appendix B
Duration of Behavior Data Sheet

Appendix C
Latency to Behavior Data Sheet

Appendix D
Data Sheet for Measuring the Intensity
of the Behavior

Appendix E
Time Sample Data Sheet

Appendix F
Permanent Products Data Sheet

Appendix G
A-B-C Data Sheet

Appendix H
Descriptive Analysis Data Sheet

Appendix I
Antecedent Manipulations Data Sheet

Appendix A   Frequency Recording Data Sheet

Behavior: _____

Definition of Behavior:

_____

_____

_____

_____

Date: _____
Observer: _____
Time Observation Starts: _____
Time Observation Ends: _____

Total Count of Behavior:

Rate of Behavior (if applicable): _____ per _____

Date: _____
Observer: _____
Time Observation Starts: _____
Time Observation Ends: _____

Total Count of Behavior:

Rate of Behavior (if applicable): _____ per _____

Date: _____
Observer: _____
Time Observation Starts: _____
Time Observation Ends: _____

Total Count of Behavior:

Rate of Behavior (if applicable): _____ per _____

Date: _____
Observer: _____
Time Observation Starts: _____
Time Observation Ends: _____

Total Count of Behavior:

Rate of Behavior (if applicable): _____ per _____

Appendix B   Duration of Behavior Data Sheet

Behavior: _____

Definition of Behavior:

_____

_____

_____

_____

_____

After each occurrence of the behavior, record the duration in the spaces provided below.
If there are more than 20 occurrences of the behavior, use a second data sheet.

Date: _____
Observer: _____
Time Observation Starts: _____
Time Observation Ends: _____

Duration 1: _____
Duration 2: _____
Duration 3: _____
Duration 4: _____
Duration 5: _____
Duration 6: _____
Duration 7: _____
Duration 8: _____
Duration 9: _____
Duration 10: _____
Duration 11: _____
Duration 12: _____
Duration 13: _____
Duration 14: _____
Duration 15: _____
Duration 16: _____
Duration 17: _____
Duration 18: _____
Duration 19: _____
Duration 20: _____

Average or Total (circle one) Duration: _____
(To calculate Average Duration, add all of the durations together and divide by the
number of occurrences of the behavior. To calculate Total Duration, add all of the
durations together.)

Appendix C   Latency to Behavior Data Sheet

Behavior: _____

Definition of Behavior:

_____

_____

_____

_____

_____

Date: _____
Observer: _____
Time Observation Starts: _____
Time Observation Ends: _____

What was the activity or stimulus?	Latency to Behavior

Average or Total (circle one) Latency: _____
(To calculate Average Latency, add all of the latencies together and divide by the number of occurrences of the behavior. To calculate Total Latency, add all of the latencies together.)

Appendix D   Data Sheet for Measuring the Intensity

Behavior: _____

Definition of Behavior:

_____

_____

_____

_____

Date: _____

Observer: _____

Time Observation Starts: _____

Time Observation Ends: _____

Intensity Level Please write in the intensity levels for this behavior.	Frequency Please make a hash mark in the box for each occurrence of the behavior at this intensity level.	Total Please add the hash marks for each level and write the total here.	Rate Divide the total by the amount of time observed.

Appendix E Time Sample Data Sheet

Behavior: _____

Definition of Behavior:

_____

_____

_____

_____

_____

Date: _____
Observer: _____
Time Observation Starts: _____
Time Observation Ends: _____
Observation Interval Length: _____
Circle which data collection procedure you are using:

      Partial Interval   Momentary Time Sample

Interval Number (If needed, write actual times next to interval number)	Did the behavior occur... ...at all if Partial Interval? ...at end of interval if Momentary Time Sample?	
1	Yes	No
2	Yes	No
3	Yes	No
4	Yes	No
5	Yes	No
6	Yes	No
7	Yes	No
8	Yes	No
9	Yes	No
10	Yes	No
11	Yes	No
12	Yes	No
13	Yes	No
14	Yes	No
15	Yes	No
16	Yes	No
17	Yes	No
18	Yes	No
19	Yes	No
20	Yes	No

(Use additional sheets if more than 20 intervals per observation.)

Total Number of "Yes": _____
(If applicable) **Percent of Intervals in which behavior occurred:** _____
("Total Yes" divided by "Total Yes" + "Total No" multiplied by 100.)

Appendix F   Permanent Products Data Sheet

Behavior: _____

Definition of Behavior:

_____

_____

_____

_____

_____

Product Measured: _____

Date: _____
Observer: _____
Time Observation Starts: _____
Time Observation Ends: _____
Total Count: _____
Rate of Behavior *(if applicable)*: _____ per _____

Date: _____
Observer: _____
Time Observation Starts: _____
Time Observation Ends: _____
Total Count: _____
Rate of Behavior *(if applicable)*: _____ per _____

Date: _____
Observer: _____
Time Observation Starts: _____
Time Observation Ends: _____
Total Count: _____
Rate of Behavior *(if applicable)*: _____ per _____

Date: _____
Observer: _____
Time Observation Starts: _____
Time Observation Ends: _____
Total Count: _____
Rate of Behavior *(if applicable)*: _____ per _____

Appendix G   A-B-C Data Sheet

Behavior: _____

Definition of Behavior:

_____

_____

_____

_____

_____

Date: _____

Observer: _____

Setting	Activity	Antecedent	Consequence	Possible function?

Possible Function 1: _____   Total Number of Occurrences: _____

Possible Function 2: _____   Total Number of Occurrences: _____

Possible Function 3: _____   Total Number of Occurrences: _____

Possible Function 4: _____   Total Number of Occurrences: _____

Possible Function 5: _____   Total Number of Occurrences: _____

Appendix H Descriptive Analysis Data Sheet

Behavior: _____

Definition of Behavior:

_____

_____

_____

_____

Date: _____
Observer: _____
Observed with: _____

For each instance of the behavior, circle the letter(s) signifying which condition(s) were in place. Use the code below:
  D=Demand   L=Low Attention   R=Restricted Access   A=Alone

Instance of the behavior?	Conditions in place?				Write intensity or duration in this space, if applicable
1	D	L	R	A	
2	D	L	R	A	
3	D	L	R	A	
4	D	L	R	A	
5	D	L	R	A	
6	D	L	R	A	
7	D	L	R	A	
8	D	L	R	A	
9	D	L	R	A	
10	D	L	R	A	
11	D	L	R	A	
12	D	L	R	A	
13	D	L	R	A	
14	D	L	R	A	
15	D	L	R	A	
16	D	L	R	A	
17	D	L	R	A	
18	D	L	R	A	
19	D	L	R	A	
20	D	L	R	A	
Total Frequencies:					
Average frequency, duration, or intensity:					

Note: For interval data, use that data sheet in conjunction with this one.

Appendix I   Antecedent Manipulations Data Sheet

Behavior: _____

Definition of Behavior:

_____

_____

_____

_____

Date:_____
Length of sessions: _____
Observer: _____
Observed with: _____

Define each condition here: _____

1)

2)

3)

4)

5)

6)

Condition	Session 1 Total	Session 2 Total	Session 3 Total	Overall Total
1)				
2)				
3)				
4)				
5)				
6)				
Which condition elicited the most target behaviors for each session?				

Index

About the Author

Beth Glasberg, Ph.D., BCBA, is a consultant for Douglass Outreach at the Douglass Developmental Disabilities Center at Rutgers, The State University of New Jersey. Beth received her Ph.D. in Clinical Psychology at Rutgers University in 1988, and has been a Board Certified Behavior Analyst since 2000. She has presented at regional, national and international conferences, and has also published several articles and book chapters. A co-author of *Siblings of Children with Autism: A Guide for Families* (Woodbine House, 2003), Beth is also a two-time recipient of the Lebec Prize for Research in Autism. Dr. Glasberg lives with her family in Princeton, New Jersey.